The Animal Connection:

Cancer and Other Diseases from Animals and Foods of Animal Origin

Agatha M. Thrash, M.D.
Calvin L. Thrash, Jr., M.D.

Yuchi Pines Institute
Seale, AL 36875

Library of Congress Cataloging in Publication Data

Thrash, Agatha M., 1931-
The animal connection.

Bibliography: p.
Includes index.
1. Cancer--Nutritional aspects. 2. Zoonosis.
3. Diseases--Causes and theories of causation.
4. Animal food--Toxicology. I. Thrash, Calvin L.,
1928- . II. Title. [DNLM: 1. Animals.
2. Neoplasms--Etiology. 3. Zoonoses. WC 950 T529a]
RC262.T48 1983 616.99'4071 82-23796
ISBN 0-942658-04-3

INTRODUCTION

The understanding of the cause of disease has passed through many phases in the history of mankind. Early in recorded history, most people felt disease was due to evil spirits. Later many physicians believed that toxicities were the cause of all illness, and most recently the idea of germs being the cause of sickness has caught on widely. Portions of all these ideas may be correct. It is certainly a fact that brain hormones resulting from such feelings as guilt, anger, anxiety, hatred, and other strong negative emotions lead to physiologic states that bring on illness. This can be thought of as evil spirits.

It is also true that various toxicities can lead to illness. Toxicities can originate outside the body or be produced inside the body from poor health habits such as overeating, eating too many varieties at a meal, failure to chew properly, and eating refined, concentrated, or junk foods.

Invasion of the body by germs can surely cause disease, particularly if the body forces are weakened and barriers are worn down by the above mentioned "evil spirits" and toxicities.

Cancer is a disease of this nature. The germ is a virus that invades the cell of a person who is weakened by poor health habits. To avoid the virus and other infectious and toxic sources of disease is the subject of this book. Most people can resist disease successfully if even two of the above three factors are functioning at a high level of efficiency.

This book grew from a study of the little publicized but rapidly mounting body of evidence that the reservoir for human cancer virus is largely in animals, those used for food as well as those kept for pets. The objective of this book is to inspire caution, to discourage the use of so much meat, milk, eggs, and cheese in the preparation of meals, and to voice concern about the close contact with pets, especially by children.

TABLE OF CONTENTS

CHAPTER ONE
Diseases Transmissible to Man From Animals and Animal Products

CAUSES OF DISEASES

Civilization is only a few short generations away from the witch doctor and the shaman in its knowledge of disease, its causation, prevention, and treatment. But in the last few years, giant strides have been made in our understanding of how man and his environment interact either to produce or prevent disease; to enjoy bountiful health or suffer dismal invalidism.

You can stay well and healthy if you work at it. By following simple practices in preventive maintenance, the very peak of cheerfulness and strength can be achieved and maintained. One of these practices is the consistent control or avoidance of sources of infection.

There are reservoirs of infection in domestic animals and livestock which impose a threat of ill-health on vast numbers of urban and rural people. Particularly is this true in tropical and sub-tropical countries. Pets as well as wildlife are potential sources of infection.

The greatest hazards, however, are presented by the consumption of eggs, meat, fish and dairy products. Diseases in food animals result in a great economic loss in the United States. If we are to feed our ever-increasing population, we must control these food losses. Animal protein in many countries is scarce even before losses from disease reduce their already dwindling food supplies. (1)

While animals are in closer contact with rural dwellers than with urban dwellers, we should bear in mind that animals play a serious role in environmental hazards in urban communities as well. Urbanization of man has at the same time concentrated the population of animals in residential areas. Approximately 60,000,000 cats and dogs share the domiciles of Americans, along with an astounding number of other "companion" animals, such as birds, monkeys, small rodents, and fish. (2)

It is suggested by Dr. James H. Steel, writing in **Laboratory Medicine,** in December, 1970 that "lower animals can serve as a source of virus strains that may cause sporadic human disease, or possible epidemics or pandemics (world-wide epidemics)". (3)

SICKNESS IN FARM AND FOOD ANIMALS

Foods used by humans come from either plants or animals. It is more likely that animal viruses are active in causing human disease than plant viruses, since plants are so biologically different from animals and humans. While plants have diseases, some of which are bacterial, some fungal, and some viral, the possibility appears quite remote that plant viruses are involved in human disease.

We do not yet know the cause of many human diseases such as arthritis, collagen disease, the wasting muscle diseases, many of the chronic and disabiling intestinal diseases (Crohn's disease, ulcerative colitis, celiac disease, and fibrocystic disease of the pancreas), many of the crippling neurological diseases, and on and on. It is not a far-fetched idea that many of these diseases of unknown cause are related to animal diseases transmitted to man either by direct contact with the animal or by ingestion of the flesh, milk, or eggs of the infected animal. (4)

Cooking does not insure that bacteria are killed. Viruses are far more resistant to destruction by heat than are bacteria. Rare roast beef reaches an internal temperature of about 60 degrees Centigrade. Even well-done roast beef may reach an internal temperature of only about 76 degrees Centigrade. Foot-and-mouth disease viruses can easily survive 80 degrees Centigrade for four hours. Frozen meats and fowl are often not cooked sufficiently to destroy all bacteria. While some diseases of animals are not shared by man, and some diseases of man cannot be contracted by animals, the transmission to man of viruses and bacteria is easily accomplished by consumption of the flesh, milk, or eggs of an infected animal. (5)

In addition to the animal diseases that man can contract because the animal itself is diseased, are diseases of humans that are transmitted because of contamination of food through carelessness of food manufacturers or handlers. While food of both plant and animal origin can be contaminated by the diseases of food handlers and food manufacturers, foods of animal origin make a better culture medium for bacteria, and a better transport medium for viruses than do foods from plant sources.

MEAT INSPECTION

Laws of meat inspection are designed to govern the sale of cattle, calves, poultry, sheep and pigs (6) sold for food. Up to the present, control has been spotty and ineffectual. Many firms shamelessly add chemicals to spoiled meats to make them look fresh.

The animal diseases present a special medical and economic challenge. They include several of the most widespread and serious infections of man. The experience of the past forty years leads us to assume that animal diseases will contribute even more to the burden of human disease in the future.

All manner of infectious diseases of animals including viral diseases, rickettsial, spirochetal, bacterial, fungal, and protozoan are common in man. Both domestic and wild animals are involved in this transmission. The list of diseases known to be communicated from animals to man is quite long (8) and is growing with each decade.

There was once a time when fish could be recommended as the most healthful of the flesh foods. This picture has changed as industrial chemicals harmful to human health have become more and more numerous and concentrated in water inhabited by fish used for food. Furthermore, human viruses present in contaminated waters are now found in fish, and can be carried to man without infecting the fish in the transaction. These organisms have been found in unprecedented numbers, and include human polio viruses, coxsackie viruses, and rheo viruses (the cause of mild respiratory infections). Coxsackie and polio viruses can be isolated from the gastrointestinal tracts of fish caught near sewer outlets from such cities as Aurora, Montgomery and Elgin along the Fox River near Chicago. One-and-one-half million people use the water system taken from the Fox River. (9)

The **News and Sun-Sentinel**, April 22, 1979 discussed a new government study showing that 14% of the dressed meat and poultry sold in supermarkets may contain chemical residues suspected of causing cancer, birth defects, toxicities, and other health problems in man. For the consumer to depend on the government inspection at slaughter houses is quite inadequate; it will not result in security against contracting common diseases of animals. (10)

To certify that a one-hundred-and-fifty pound human did not die of a communicable disease may take a highly trained pathologist an hour or two of inspection in the autopsy room and a week or two of study of microscope slides and chemical and bacterial testing. Yet, a few years back, the average meat inspector was spending only eight seconds per 1500-pound carcass. Often, the meat was consumed before the inspector could have gotten reports from a laboratory even if test samples had been obtained at the time of the eight second examination. It is unlikely that the situation is any better today.

ANTIBIOTICS IN ANIMAL FEED

For reasons not yet known, antibiotics fed to animals increase their rate of growth and reduce the total quantity of food necessary for the animal to reach full maturity. Almost half of the antibiotics produced in America go into animal feed. There are, however, serious problems for the well-being of man in this practice. One of these problems is the development of resistance by the germ to the antibiotic used; they simply learn to live in an environment containing antibiotics without being inhibited in growth. (11)

CHAPTER TWO
Chickens, Pigs, Fish and Bees

POULTRY AND EGGS

It has been suspected for several decades that human leukemia is related to the leukosis of chickens, but no definite evidence could be obtained. A report appeared in 1971 of a study demonstrating the resemblance between the lysozymes (enzymes which fight microorganisms) found in human leukemia and those found in egg whites. (12) A further incrimination of eggs in human cancer production is found in the demonstration of a cancer-producing activity from the growth factor of egg yolks. Its potential relationship to cancers of humans is discussed in a 1960 report in **Neoplasma.** (13)

That eggs do not represent the best food for man even apart from the transmission of disease germs is illustrated by the fact that a large number of allergies are produced by the use of eggs in humans. Bladder allergies resembling cystitis, urethritis, various skin inflammations, gastrointestinal symptoms, and even conjunctival allergies (reddening of the eyes), occur as a result of eating eggs. (14) When egg white is injected into the peritoneal space of rats, there follows swelling of the paws, nose, tongue, and loss of blood pressure. It is assumed to be due to the release of histamine or histamine-like substances. These chemicals are known to be produced in allergic type reactions. (15)

A cerebral food allergy has been ascribed to eggs in which transient loss of vision occurs, along with headache, hives, and other symptoms. In addition to this, there was reported a type of reaction to eggs that consisted of vertigo, temporary loss of vision, headaches, and partial amnesia (loss of memory). The attacks stopped when eggs were removed from the diet. (16)

Many gastrointestinal problems, one of which is infectious diarrhea, are related to chickens and eggs. A 14-year-old boy who had spent four days plucking chickens at a farm, developed watery diarrhea, abdominal pain, and mucus. Both the pigs and the chickens on the farm showed **Campylobacter,** a germ capable of causing diarrhea. The origin of the boy's diarrhea was definitely diagnosed when his own stools showed the same **Campylobacter.** (17)

The maintenance of chickens in crowded and unsanitary conditions compounds the problems caused by infection. Shipping great distances for sale and slaughter makes chickens highly susceptible to epizootic spread of bacterial and other infectious diseases. In the livestock industry, the producer is entirely free to add antibiotics in whatever quantity and whatever kind he wishes without even consulting a veterinarian or health professional.

Most meat, including chickens, bought by consumers is heavily contaminated by intestinal microorganisms from the animals, chiefly **E. coli.** If the chickens have been fed antibiotics, these germs are usually resistant to antibiotics. Both the livestock and the pharmaceutical interests have waged a continual lobbying campaign in an effort to prevent government control of this situation. These commercial interests do not admit the health hazards involved from these practices. (18) **Salmonella** in eggs is often reported. (19, 20)

In addition to antibiotics and contagious infections, sometimes chickens are subjected to contaminated feed. Chickens and eggs were contaminated by polychlorinated biphenyls in Idaho and Montana in 1979. (21) This type of contamination can expose hundreds of thousands of people to toxic chemicals in a few hours. Such a situation is almost impossible to control, as the human exposure usually occurs before the opportunity for detection.

DISEASES FROM PORK AND PORK PRODUCTS

Trichinosis may be forgotten, but it is not gone. In Louisiana in the late winter of 1979, there were nineteen cases of trichinosis reported during a six-week period The mean incubation period was seventeen days with a range of 5 to 31 days. The people experienced fever, muscle aching, and swelling around the eyes. Trichinosis is generally not recognized, and probably produces these non-specific symptoms thousands of times for each time they are correctly diagnosed and reported to the health department. Seven out of ten people who use pork products have antibodies to Trichina organisms in their bloodstream. Yet, the vast majority of these people are unaware of ever having had a Trichina infection. Much of just feeling bad, poor performance, and loss of physical drive may be due to long-term infestation with Trichina. For the rest of life, the person continues to receive doses of inflammatory products and waste material from the Trichina worms encysted in the most active muscle groups, such as the diaphragm. He produces antibodies to them, which diverts some of his strength from vital functions, and contributes to the loss of sense of well-being.

It is unlikely that most individuals suffering from diseases they contracted from the use of animal products or their exposure to pets or livestock ever correctly identify the true origin of the disease. In one outbreak, there were 31 people who ate smoked sausage, but only 19 of them became ill, and that after many days. (22) The long incubation period and the fact that not everyone who eats a product comes down with the disease, adds to the difficulty in making the association of the disease with its animal origin.

Between 1968 and 1975, fifteen cases of meningitis or septicemia due to a special type of Streptococcus, the group R Streptococcus, were reported among meat handlers. Two of the men died. (23) Men who work in pork processing industries may get this serious neurologic disease which can leave them with deafness and unsteadiness. Hotdogs are a potential source of a type of organism causing sporotrichosis, a skin disease characterized by a string of nodules developing upward along the path of the lymphatics. (24)

FISH

In Michigan and several other areas, **Diphyllobothrium latum**, the fish tapeworm, has been identified in man. Opportunity for infection occurs when undercooked fish is eaten. A 51-year-old man passed a long, whitish string which he took to his physician. He had had no bowel complaints, but reported a fishing trip to the Northwest area eleven months before. The fish tapeworm normally lives in the small intestine of fish in subarctic and temperate regions. It is the largest tapeworm found in man. It competes with the host for nutrients, which is the major cause for disability produced in man. Especially notable is megaloblastic anemia due to vitamin B-12 deficiency since the tapeworm inhabits the part of the small bowel where B-12 is absorbed. Numbness of the extremities is the most common complaint, along with fatigue, weakness, and dizziness. (25) All of these are vague and non-specific complaints and can go on for years before the appropriate diagnosis is suspected.

BEES AND HONEY

Bees have only recently been recognized as a cause of disease in humans. The virus which causes acute bee paralysis has properties similar to those of picornaviruses, the name given to a group of small RNA viruses which belong to the enteroviruses and the rhinoviruses. They cause intestinal and upper respiratory diseases, respectively. Foot-and-mouth virus of cattle and encephalomyocarditis of rodents, along with certain plant and insect viruses belong to this group. For many people, the diseases caused by this group of viruses are minor fevers, although some of these viruses are responsible for epidemics. There have been no known human diseases from acute bee paralysis virus, but its existence among bees should be recognized.

Botulism from honey has been reported in infants under the age of six months, but not in children over six months. The disease is usually difficult to diagnose and is very dangerous. Symptoms of infant botulism are profound weakness and inability of the infant to suck and swallow. The cry becomes feeble, and there may be loss of head control. Of nine infants having botulism, six were principally breast-fed. However, all infants had been exposed to some additional food before the onset of their symptoms. (26) Other symptoms of infant botulism include dehydration and failure to thrive. Some have believed that botulism is related to the sudden infant death syndrome. (27) Other sources of botulism have been home canned, low-acid vegetables that have not been recooked before serving (10 to 20 minutes required to inactivate the toxin). Canned fish, or their eggs, and canned mushrooms not recooked have been known to produce botulism symptoms in adults. The symptoms of botulism include double vision, abdominal pain, nausea, and vomiting.

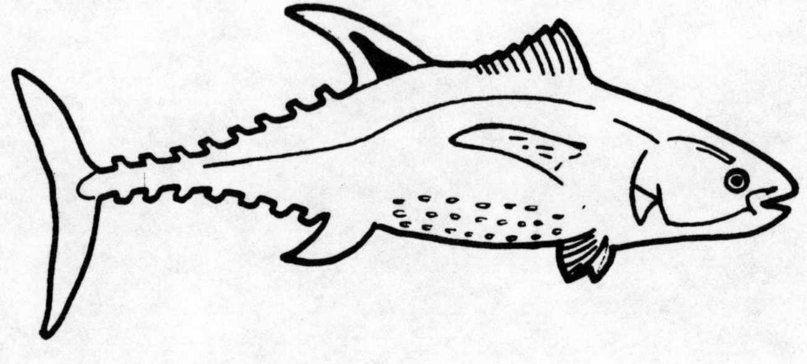

CHAPTER THREE
Some Specific Diseases Obtained From Animals

Over 100 human diseases can be acquired from animals. A few of these will be discussed in this chapter.

SKIN DISEASES IN ANIMALS

A number of animal diseases have the manifestation of itching which may be relieved by the animal through scratching, rubbing, rolling, nibbling, head shaking, licking, feather-picking, cannibalism, baldness, thickening of the skin, loss of the outer layer of skin, exuberance in the animal, or bleeding into the skin. Man may contract diseases from domestic animals having itching as a symptom. These include erysipelas, brucellosis, ringworm, lice, mites, scabies, and papular urticaria (small itching skin lesions). (28)

SALMONELLOSIS AND OTHER DISEASES CAUSING DIARRHEA

Salmonellosis (food poisoning) is a disease characterized by diarrhea, chills, fever, abdominal pain, and sometimes prostration and death. The symptoms may begin anywhere from 7 to 72 hours after eating eggs, poultry or dairy products. (29) Frozen, fresh, or dried egg products can cause salmonellosis. (30, 31) Practically all eggs contain bacteria. Salmonella germs enter the egg in the oviduct at an immature stage. The wide occurrence of ovarian infection in domestic fowl has come about only in the last few years.

Most cases of salmonellosis do not come to medical attention, and are usually passed off as a cold or flu. A cooking temperature of 350 degrees for thirty minutes is recommended to kill the germ. (32) In one report in 1979, twenty-three patients with Salmonella were reported by the Atlanta based Center for Disease Control (CDC), ranging from ages 6 months to 59 years, the median age being 11 years. Sixteen were female, seven were male. Thirteen lived in one city, nine in another, and one in an area midway between the two cities. Twelve of the patients attended school, but no school had more than four cases. Ninety-one per cent of the patients had fever, and eighty-seven percent had abdominal pain. Nausea and vomiting were also prominent symptoms. Both low fat and whole milk had been consumed by the patients reported by the Center for Disease Control. (33) Salmonellosis has been associated with the consumption of non-fat powdered milk which apparently served as the vehicle in some cases. (34, 35)

Horses are a common source of salmonella infection in man. In one study, 42% of horses used for pleasure riding were found to be "asymptomatic shedders" of Salmonella germs. Those who frequent the riding stable may pick up the disease-producing germ and either develop the disease or become asymptomatic carriers. The type of Salmonella obtained from horses is the third most common type of Salmonella cultured from humans in the United States. (36)

Pet turtles are a well-known source of Salmonella. This includes those certified to be Salmonella-free! (37, 38, 39) Many humans are carriers of Salmonella and can infect birds, turkeys, ducks, and chickens. (40) Feces and urine carry the germs. Humans can get salmonellosis from contact with infected cattle. Salmonellosis in man and animals continues to be an ever-increasing problem. (41)

An epidemic of gastrointestinal diseases caused by chocolate milk was found to be due to **Yersinia enterocolitica.** (42)

STAPHYLOCOCCI

Food poisoning from milk and animal products can be caused by Staphylococcus toxin, which produces acute gastroenteritis with severe abdominal cramps and collapse, beginning one to six hours after the ingestion of ham, creamy pastries, cheese, milk products, potato salad, or custards. (43) These foods are favored growth places for staphylococci.

There are many infectious diseases that are still transmitted by cattle. In the past such diseases as anthrax, cowpox, brucellosis, foot-

and-mouth disease, rabies, actinomycosis, ringworm, herpes, tetanus, gas gangrene, parasites, scarlet fever, diptheria, streptococcal sore throat, and polio have been transmitted to man by cattle or through milk. Milk-borne epidemics of infectious disease are an historical fact and are probably much more involved in present epidemics than is recognized. (44)

BRUCELLOSIS

Although less common now than formerly, brucellosis remains a disease transmissible from cattle to man, even after decades of serious attempts to eradicate the disease from cattle. (45) In cattle it causes sterility, slow breeding, and abortion. (46) In Brazil, eight percent of dairy herds have brucellosis. (47) Brucellosis is a disease obtained from farm animals, cattle, goats, hogs, sheep or dogs. It is called Bang's disease in cattle, and undulant fever in man. Anyone can get brucellosis, but men have it four times as frequently as women, probably because men work more around livestock, in packing houses, dairies, meat shops, and as veterinarians.

Brucellosis is obtained fairly easily from an animal, but rarely, if ever, from another person. It can be acquired by handling raw meats, drinking unpasteurized milk, eating dairy products made from unpasteurized milk, assisting in the delivery of young animals, or breathing dust carrying the germs, especially around barnyards, and slaughter houses.

The symptoms, much like flu, last much longer. Weakness, headache, fever that goes up and down, chills, heavy sweats, joint pains, backache, loss of weight, and poor appetite are all symptoms. Even after a person seems well of the acute symptoms there may be a recurrence of symptoms months or even years later, and a persistent feeling of being "not up to par." The fever and malaise may increase to debilitation in some patients, with periods of being worse and periods of being better. There is no known medical cure, although hydrotherapy has been reported to be very beneficial in undulant fever. Individuals who work with infected herds or who drink unpasteurized milk are most subject to brucellosis.

The incidence of brucellosis in the United States has declined since 1947 when 6,321 cases were reported. Only 175 cases were reported in 1973, but there were indications of a subsequent rise in incidence as 247 and 328 cases were reported respectively in 1974 and 1975. Disease is again occurring in states that had previously been free of the disease, and there is an increased incidence of the disease in states in which brucellosis has never been eradicated in animals. (48)

STREPTOCOCCI

Sore throat caused by bacteria has been repeatedly linked to milk. (49, 50) The principal type of sore throat linked to milk-drinking is streptococcal sore throat. Dr. Frank Oski, in the book, **Don't Drink Your Milk,** reports the experience of a prominent pediatrician who has not seen a case of streptococcal sore throat in a child who did not give a history of consuming milk in the previous five day period. (51)

Another streptococcus (**Streptococcus bovis**- from cows, a group D streptococcus) previously thought to be sensitive to penicillin is now known to be not sensitive to the antibiotic, making it difficult to treat by ordinary methods. This streptococcus is a cause of endocarditis, a life-threatening disease of the heart valves. (52)

A veterinarian reviewing the various diseases communicable from cattle to man describes them under three main headings as follows: Infections primarily of animal origin; infections in which the disease germ produces primarily human diseases; and infections in which the cow is a passive carrier, the germ being a contaminant in food products. Germs causing sore throat can fall in any of these three categories.

Nanna Svartz, a distinguished Swedish researcher, has presented evidence accumulated over a thirty year span, to incriminate a streptococcus in the etiology of rheumatoid arthritis. The organism is found in milk, and is not destroyed by pasteurization. (54)

HEPATITIS

Oysters were associated with seven cases of hepatitis in Mobile, Alabama and three cases in

Albany, Georgia. (55) In 1955 an epidemic of hepatitis involving over 600 people in Goteburg, Sweden, was traced to consumption of raw oysters. (56)

Significant outbreaks related to contaminated shellfish have been reported from the Pascagoula River of Mississippi and from the Raritan, Chesapeake and Narragansett Bay areas of New England. A study of Koff (57) concluded that raw shellfish consumption may account for a sizeable incidence of the hepatitis seen in sporadic, or non-epidemic, cases in New England.

NEWCASTLE DISEASE

This is a disease transmissible to man from pets and poultry. It also causes a respiratory disease in fowl. The virus spreads quickly to birds. Exotic Newcastle disease can kill highly susceptible birds even before symptoms appear. If the bird does have symptoms they usually consist of unsteadiness, heavy breathing, and a mucous discharge. Birds have been known to carry the virus for as long as 400 days and yet not come down with the disease themselves. Even healthy and robust birds can be dangerous carriers. (58)

In man, the disease results in severe conjunctivitis involving usually only one eye, rarely both. It is interesting to note that the virulence of Newcastle disease virus is diminished when the virus passes through chickens kept on a diet deficient in vitamin B-2. Vitamin B-12, however, has no direct influence on virus pathogenicity. (59) It may be that some human infections behave similarly by having less virulence in the presence of low levels of vitamin B-12.

LEPTOSPIROSIS

Leptospirosis is characterized by any of the following symptoms: fever, sore eyes, muscle aches, meningitis, kidney impairment, a rash, and occasionally jaundice. It can be obtained from the urine of infected dogs, pigs, and other animals. Patients may become prostrate. Usually they recover within ten to fourteen days without treatment. About 31 percent of cases are traced to contact with rats; 30 percent with dogs; 21 percent with cattle; and 13 percent with swine. (60)

It is widely believed that apparently healthy, immunized dogs are safe to be around. This is not true, and exposure to pets can end fatally. Many times, healthy dogs can excrete Leptospirosis in their urine. (61) A case of leptospirosis in a pregnant woman is reported. It was first thought to be influenza with fever and headache, but it resulted in the death of her fetus. (62)

Once while we were presenting a series of lectures in a college town, a lady who listened to one of our lectures on animal diseases sent up a note after one of the evening sessions. The note read as follows: "The death of my daughter and near death of my son (my husband and I were also sick) we attribute to a disease our dog had -leptospirosis. The symptoms in my son were identical to those in our dog. The diagnosis in the dog was made by a veterinarian."

MULTIPLE SCLEROSIS

Between 1938 and 1942, a group of workers who had been involved in a veterinary research project came down with "disseminated sclerosis" (multiple sclerosis). They had all worked with swayback and other nerve diseases of lambs. The patients all died young, before the age of 55, and at the time of death had had the neurological disease for twelve to twenty years. One patient developed acute retrobulbar neuritis and lost the vision in the right eye. Two cases had duodenal ulcers for which surgery was performed. In one case, the sister of a patient who died also developed multiple sclerosis. (63)

ALZHEIMER'S DISEASE

A study reported in **Internal Medicine News** (64) suggests that Alzheimer's disease, a form of senile dementia, may be caused by an infective agent. Other reports suggest that the effect of a viral agent superimposed on a hereditary susceptibility can cause various forms of dementia, leukemia, and Down's syndrome. Although the report draws no link with the use of animal products in the diet, any reservoir of viruses would be suspect.

FOOT-AND-MOUTH DISEASE

This disease is an acute, very contagious, viral disease of wild and domestic animals which is communicable to man. It is characterized by blisters on the lips, oral cavity, pharynx, legs and feet. Milk has been implicated as a vehicle for the transmission of this disease.

The virus survives pasturization of milk. Cream, in particular, offers a marked protective effect for this virus. It enables the virus to withstand heating at ninety-three degrees Centigrade for sixteen seconds. This temperature is in excess of that of commercial processing, and pasteurization is unable to kill this virus. (65, 66)

CATS, DOGS, AND OTHER HOUSE PETS

Generally speaking, cats are more likely than dogs to spread disease to children and household members. Furthermore, cats, more than other pets, spread disease to dogs and other companion animals. Cats are a threat to humans by their many diseases, including rabies. Cat bites, scratches, or fleas from cats may transmit several kinds of infection.

One of the most serious and widespread diseases from cats is toxoplasmosis. Toxoplasma antibodies are common in human blood serum indicating a previous infection with toxoplasma organisms. In adults the symptoms may be mild and resemble "flu." A regular occurrence is chorioretinitis (blindness) in children of mothers who were apparently infected during pregnancy. Toxoplasmosis also causes mental retardation, hydrocephalus, eye diseases, deformities, and other neurological disorders that may not become apparent until after childhood.

Fetal death in late pregnancy or the newborn period is a frequent result of toxoplasma infection in the mother. Toxoplasma may also be contracted by eating raw or inadequately cooked meat,and from several kinds of livestock and pets. It is notable and probably highly significant that Eskimos have no cats and no toxoplasmosis.

Different from Toxoplasma is Toxocara, the common roundworm of most dogs and cats. When humans are infested with these worms, they produce a disease called visceral larva migrans. The child comes down with very ordinary symptoms of bronchitis, fever, enlarged liver, and some pneumonia. Many cases are passed off as the flu or a cold. This makes the true incidence in man nearly impossible to determine. The eosinophil count in the blood is sometimes high. (Eosinophils are white blood cells which become more numerous in the blood of persons having allergies and infestations with parasites.) While the disease is generally mild, it tends to hang on for a few months. Occasionally there have been fatalities reported. The dog or cat hookworm can cause cutaneous larva migrans or creeping eruption, an intensely itchy skin disease from which patients generally recover without any treatment. (67, 68)

A two-year-old boy began to feel bad with a runny nose and fever. In a very short time, he developed cough and paleness. He started to lose weight. He was given a large number of drugs including Dimetapp, ampicillin, theophylline, and dexamethasone. His white cell count was 19,000 with 44 percent eosinophils (normal is 0 to 3). The family had recently acquired a new puppy and had had a cat for several years. Roundworm and tapeworm ova were found in the puppy. A sister who had played with the puppy also had a runny nose which had been diagnosed as "allergic rhinitis." The child was tested for Toxocara by the usual tests (indirect hemagglutination and bentonite flocculation titers to Toxocara) and found to be negative. But when the boy's serum was tested for specific antibodies for Toxocara, he was found to have a very high titer, diagnostic for the dog and cat roundworm. He recovered after a few weeks of illness. (69)

About half of all dogs and cats harbor **Pasteurella multocida,** a germ causing redness, swelling, pain, and tenderness beginning a few hours after receiving a cat or dog bite. It will eventually develop abscesses and hard, red flesh around the bite with enlarged lymph nodes in the nearby areas. The disease may spread to produce hemorrhagic septicemia (blood poisoning), osteomyelitis, and meningitis.

Cat scratch fever can be obtained from a cat or dog scratch, a bite of an animal, or from a rose thorn scratch from roses grown in places where cats play. In the area of the scratch, there is a blister which leads to an ulcer. A fever develops and the nearby lymph nodes enlarge and sometimes open up and drain pus. Patients recover without treatment in a few weeks or months.

Rheumatoid arthritis patients have been shown to have had greater exposure to sick animals than did control patients. This suggests that pets may serve as a reservoir for infectious agents causing rheumatoid arthritis. (53)

DISEASES FROM OTHER ANIMALS

Psittacosis, a pulmonary disease with fever, shortness of breath, cough and other respiratory tract symptoms can be contracted from birds. The mortality rate is 5 to 10 percent. Patients often do not suspect they have caught a disease from birds. Pet hamsters have been the source of an outbreak of lymphocytic choriomeningitis, a disease characteristically producing a fever, headache, and severe muscle aches.

Histoplasmosis, a fungus disease causing symptoms that range from insignificant to fatal, can be acquired particularly from exposure to infected flocks in the chicken houses. Two hundred thousand new cases are expected to occur every year in America.

Other diseases from animals include vesicular stomatitis, and pox virus. Herpes viruses are found in all animal species, including birds. Influenza of man and swine flu are biologically related. The 1918-1919 influenza outbreak in both humans and hogs were simultaneous. The disease was caused by the combined activity of **Hemophilus influenza suis** and a filterable virus. The disease made its first appearance in autumn of 1918. The serum of most humans born after 1918 contains antibodies to swine flu; those born before 1918 have no antibodies. Epidemics began explosively in October or November, and were usually finished by March. The Hong Kong flu virus, first identified in man in 1968, is antigenically related to an influenza virus first isolated from horses in 1963, and is thought to be the same virus.

Newborn infants may contract listeriosis, a disease that causes fever during pregnancy, but is usually undiagnosed. The baby gets the germ during passage through the birth canal or is infected from environmental sources. (70) Cows, goats, sheep, hogs, poultry (especially turkeys), fish, crabs, and rabbits are known reservoirs of the disease.

Monkeys are no friends of humans. They are dangerous pets and can transmit measles, encephalitis (Arboviruses), amoebic dysentery, and many other serious illnesses. Hemorrhagic disease of monkeys begins as a severe case of feeling bad followed by impaired consciousness, headache, high fever, vomiting, diarrhea and a rash on the skin and inside the mouth. The eyes become red and sore and the lymph nodes become swollen. There is bleeding into many tissues and body openings with signs of involvement of both the central and peripheral nerves. About one-third of the cases die! (71) Monkeys can also transmit tuberculosis and hepatitis. Fifty documented cases of hepatitis are mentioned in a single report. (72)

It has been suggested that systemic lupus erythematosus is a disease of animals transmitted to man. However, a test on eleven dogs of patients who had systemic lupus failed to support the hypothesis that lupus is a disease of animals. (73) Nevertheless, the implication is not banished by the results of this one report. Further studies on the relationship of lupus to animal disease are urgently needed.

Non-human reservoirs for human cholera exist in cows, goats, dogs, and chickens. These reservoirs in animals may serve as sources of infection in humans. (74)

DISEASES FROM WILD ANIMALS

A large number of diseases are transmitted from wild animals. Dogs were once the principal source of human rabies, but during the past two decades, wild animals such as the bat, skunk, fox and raccoon have been the principal sources. In recent years, fewer than five cases of human rabies have been reported in the United States per year.

The bobcat has been discovered to be the carrier in a case of human plague. Eighteen cases of human plague occurred in the United States in 1980. (75) A 25-year-old rancher began having headaches, chills, and fever progressing to vomiting and a massive swelling in the left armpit. He had cut his left hand shortly before skinning a bobcat. The patient died a few days later.

Rocky Mountain spotted fever is thought to be primarily an infection of wild rodents spread to man by several species of ticks. This includes both wood and dog ticks.

The reservoir for the protozoan **Giardia lamblia**, which is a common cause of diarrhea, weight loss, and intestinal malabsorption, is now felt to be both wild and domesticated animals. The beaver has been definitely implicated, and dogs and other animals are suspected.

ANIMAL PRODUCTS SUCH AS BONE MEAL

Imported bone meal is the only material to which the general public is exposed potentially infected with anthrax . Infected bone meal is incorporated in the feed of animals, and bone meal is sometimes used as a fertilizer in agriculture. (76)

It is difficult to know how many infections are exchanged between man and his animal domestics. Recent figures indicate that 130 to 150 major and 80 to 90 minor diseases are shared by man and animals. Years ago, Ralph Nader said that at least 30 diseases were considered transmissible to man through meat, milk, poultry, eggs, and other foods of animal origin.

From the material presented in this chapter it can be readily discerned that there is no safety in owning domesticated animals, and that animal products are a hazard in the diet of humans.

CHAPTER FOUR
The Relation Between Milk, Eggs, and Other Animal Products and Cancer

CAUSES OF CANCER

Cancer undoubtedly begins with a single cell. The cell escapes from the regulatory mechanisms of the body, perhaps by a basic change in the way DNA of the nucleus is formed. Somehow, there develops a changed relation of the cancer cell with neighboring cells of the body, a change thought to be due to the electrical surface charges of the cell, its electrical polarity, and the cell chemistry. (77) Electrical charges on the surface of cells may account for both uncontrolled growth and improper cell movement. "The electrical voltage which normally exists across the surface membrane acts to exert precise control over division in body cells." (78)

In embryonic life when cells are migrating to find their natural positions, and in repair of tissue when there is scar formation, division and movement of cells occur until one cell bumps against another. At that moment, "contact inhibition" stops cell division and movement. As long as the majority of cells in an area remain strong and possess good contact inhibition, even if one cell should become cancerous, it can be kept in check for years, or even an entire lifetime by the natural barriers imposed against the cancer. But, as often happens, the resistance of all cells becomes reduced by poor health habits, retention of waste products, or formation of toxins, and the cancer cell finds no barrier to its migration and multiplication.

Cells such as nerve and muscle, that are usually non-dividing, have high negative membrane voltages--on the order of minus 90 millivolts. Those cells such as the lining cells of the digestive tract, that divide routinely, have lower voltages. Tumor cells are much lower, having voltages in the minus 10 millivolt range. High negative voltages block cell division by preventing synthesis of DNA (deoxyribonucleic acid), an essential component of the nucleus. Thus, a reduction in negative voltage across the membrane, and a corresponding inhibition of DNA synthesis fits with the characteristics of abnormal cell division.

Infection neutralizes contact inhibition, and in many virus infections there is loss of controlled cell growth and motion. (79) Eating excessive fats alters the surface charge of cells. Free fats in the blood stream cause clumping of red blood cells. The presence of alcohol in the blood also causes clumping of red blood cells. This clumping reduces tissue nutrition and oxygenation, as the clusters of red blood cells cannot flow freely through the capillaries, and the microcirculation in vital areas is slowed severely. All of these factors--virus infections, excessive fats, and alcohol in the blood--are known to increase one's likelihood of developing cancer.

More than 85 viruses are known to cause cancers in animals. Of the 31 adenoviruses isolated from man, twelve are known to cause cancer in animals. More than a dozen viruses that primarily cause leukemia have been identified. Virus-like particles have been found in cases of dog, mouse, human, and cattle leukemia.

The Epstein-Barr (EB) virus was first discovered in 1964, in cells cultured from Burkitt's lymphoma, a malignant tumor of children which is at home in certain areas of Africa and New Guinea. (80) Since 1964, there has been accumulating evidence that this virus is indeed the causative agent of Burkitt's lymphoma. A herpes virus, indistinguishable from the EB virus, has been shown to cause Marek's disease, a malignant lymphoma of chickens. The infection is also carried in the eggs. A vaccine has been made for chickens which prolongs the life of the chickens, but unfortunately does not reduce the transmission of the virus.

CANCER IS TRANSMISSIBLE

Cancer is not considered a contagious disease in the strictest sense, but through the years, evidence has mounted that cancer is at least slightly transmissible, possibly from human to human as in cancer of the cervix from herpes virus, but especially from animals to humans as in leukemias and lymphomas.

In addition to the venereal spread of herpes viruses, they are also known to be present in various dairy products including "sterile" milk, raw milk, and chocolate milk. Cancer-producing viruses actually demonstrated to resist pasteurization temperatures are Rauscher and Moloney murine leukemia viruses, Moloney and Rous sarcoma viruses, adenovirus 12, herpes simplex virus, and reovirus 1 (not considered a cancer-producing virus, but may somehow assist in the cancerous process as they are found in human lymphomas and cat leukemia). (81) Lip and cervical cancers show reactions to antibodies made with herpes simplex virus antigens obtained from animal cells infected with herpes simplex virus, giving evidence in favor of the possibility that this virus causes both lip and cervical cancer. Normal human cells do not react with the antibodies.

Indefinite statements are often expressed concerning identifying a certain cancer virus in humans by the antibodies produced in an animal. We show no such insecurity with other viruses: why should we do so with cancer viruses? If we find antibodies to smallpox virus or measles virus in an animal we confidently say the animal has had the human infection of smallpox or measles. But when a cancer virus stimulates an antibody response in an animal we do not confidently state that the animal was infected by that particular virus. It is as if we are afraid to say that the virus that caused cancer in the cow or dog is the same virus that produces an identical antibody in humans.

For years, conclusions in regard to cancer have been held back by reluctance to accept the evidence of antibodies. It was not until 1981 that definite statements were made in medical literature declaring that the cause of leukemia in humans is "an RNA agent similiar to those causing leukemia in animals but never before clearly tied to the condition in man." (82) Investigation in the field of animal viruses related to human cancer has been strangely neglected, considering the prominent position animal products have in the marketplace, and pets have at the fireside.

THE HELPER VIRUS

It is now understood that a relatively harmless virus may serve as a "helper virus" to activate a potentially dangerous one to induce cancer. A number of virus diseases transmitted by animals could be used by cancer viruses as "helper viruses." Other viruses are sometimes required in order to help a cancer virus of the ribonucleic acid (RNA, an essential component of cells) or DNA types to produce an actual cancer in an animal. In 1972, **The Journal of the American Medical Association** (83) carried this statement: "Although some viruses, which may occur widely in food and water, are not considered to be pathologic for man, it has been speculated that when they infect an unnatural host, such as man, they may play a role in carcinogenesis" (cancer production).

IS THE VIRUS IDEA NEW TO CANCER?

There is increasing evidence that cancer viruses are spread through the same process as other infectious diseases. For more than sixty years it has been known that viruses induce cancer in chickens, and it has been around forty years since virus-caused tumors in animals were first discovered.

To transform a cell from normal to cancerous, one method a virus uses is that the protein coat of the virus first dissolves in the cell membrane of the victim cell. Then the coat opens up and becomes one with the cell membrane, about like adding a link to a chain. Next, the particle containing the genes, the genome DNA or RNA, is released into the cell, a process called viropexis. The virus particle then acts as independent genetic material inside the host cells using the cell's own mechanisms to reproduce itself abundantly. This particle may remain a part of the genetic information in the nucleus of the cells, even when the virus itself can no longer be detected in the daughter cells, as it is lying dormant to be activated by radiation, excessive fats, a carcinogen, or something else, at some later time or future generation.

The DNA viruses include polyoma virus, simian, adenoviruses, herpes virus, and pox viruses. Two herpes viruses are associated with forms of human cancer. (84) Both types of viruses multiply within the host cells and produce antigens. The Bittner cancer viruses of mouse milk have been seen by the use of the electron microscope. Newly born mice pups taken from their mothers and put with mothers having no virus particles have one-fourth the cancer of those fed by their natural mothers. (85) (See also Appendix A)

In one study, a virus that caused cancer of the breast in women produced an antigen close to, or identical with, the antigen produced by the virus causing breast cancer in mice. (86) It is also very similar or identical to a monkey virus which causes breast cancer in monkeys. (87) It is quite possible that further testing will prove breast cancer viruses in all species to be identical.

VIRUS IN MILK, BLOOD, OR FLESH

In mice, the concentration of the cancer virus in milk is equal to that in the mammary gland itself, suggesting that the virus is multiplying rapidly during the time of milk production. These results show that as far as viral transmission is concerned, **milk is as good a source of material for cancer virus as is the blood or flesh of an animal.** (88)

Virus-like particles are found in breast milk of other animals and humans having cancer of the breast. (89) A marker enzyme, RNA-dependent DNA polymerase, also called reverse transcriptase, has been found in all animal cancer-producing RNA viruses. It has also been identified in many of the human milk viral particles and breast tissue samples of human breast cancer victims, suggesting a common origin. (90)

Some portions of genetic material found in virus particles from human milk are identical to those found in known animal RNA cancer viruses. (91)

CANCER AND CONTACT WITH ANIMALS

We live in a very unfortunate time of earth's history. The most desirable place to rear children is in rural areas, and a valuable method of training children to shoulder responsibility is by giving them animals to care for. Yet at the present time the hazards of contact with animals are increasing. There is a statistically significant association between farming and death from leukemia and multiple myeloma. (92) Virus particles with diameters approximately 60 to 110 mu were detected in concentrated milk from cows in a herd with a high incidence of lymphosarcoma. Even those herds apparently lymphosarcoma-free showed virus particles in pooled tank samples of milk (93) indicating that the absence of physical signs in the cow **does not insure** the milk to be free of viruses. Although it has not yet been proven in the laboratory, leukemia in cattle is assumed by many authorities in cattle diseases to be transmitted from mother to offspring by means of colostrum and milk. (94, 95) There is a need for work to be done along these lines to establish the safety (or lack of it) of milk, as milk continues to be certified to be safe for children and older people to drink. (See also Appendix B)

Two chimpanzees at the Yerkes Regional Primate Research Center of Emory University died of a type of pneumonia, rare in humans, and unknown previously in chimpanzees. The two chimpanzees were on a special diet--milk from a herd of cows having a high incidence of lymphosarcoma, and having virus-like particles in their milk. The researchers were trying to determine the significance of these virus-like particles revealed by electron microscopy. The rare type of pneumonia was caused by **Pneumocystis carinii**, a type of pneumonia almost always associated in humans with leukemia or other malignancies, or in persons with some sort of immune deficiency. The question is raised as to whether or not this rare type of pneumonia is acquired in humans at the same time the viral agent for leukemia and other malignancies is acquired. (96)

A group of researchers noted that while they were trying to produce hardening of the arteries in rats by prolonged feeding of milk and egg yolk, the rats developed tumors in various parts of the body, particularly in the liver. It was understood by the researchers that the tumors were the result of the milk and egg diet. (97)

The association between farming as an occupation and leukemia has been recognized for years. The association is strongest for men under age 60 with lymphatic and the acute types of leukemia. Poultry farmers are especially hard-hit, having the highest proportion of excess cases as determined by a study of death certificates in Washington state. (98)

CANCER INCIDENCE RISING

Trends of deaths from breast cancer in the United States have been rising since 1910. The breast cancer rates per 100,000 in all ages, in 1911 was 7.5; in 1920 it was 8.8; in 1930, 11.2; in 1964-1965 it was 21.55. Similarly animals have shown a great increase during the same period. Known animal RNA breast cancer viruses are identical to certain RNA particles found in one-third of human milk samples furnishing further evidence that human and animal milk carry **identical cancer viruses.** (99) The milk of leukemic cattle is a very rich source of virus particles. "It is tempting to consider milk as a possible vehicle for the transmission of a leukemia virus..." (100) The viruses are present in cattle for years before the animal develops the disease. Cattle lymphoma is capable of spreading from one animal to another, and from one herd to another. There is also vertical transmission from cow to calf. In children, the age of three to four is the period of peak incidence of leukemia deaths; (101) milk-drinking is heaviest in humans during and preceding these years.

Other RNA viruses cause polio, colds, and influenza. They replicate without DNA, and the genetic material is translated into protein. We agree with the researchers who say that there is unmistakable evidence that the virus RNA from human cancer is identical to the virus RNA that causes similar tumors in animals. (102) There may be both horizontal (person-to-person) and vertical (parent-to-child) transmission of cancer viruses. (103) It is easily recognized that some types of malignancies "run in families." There has also been reported the phenomenon of clustering of cancer cases. This occurrence of multiple cancer cases in a small group or geographic area surely suggsts a shared environment or food supply as the source of the cancer; it further strongly implicates an infectious agent as the cause of cancer, leaving little doubt that the agent is a virus. We believe all cancers are caused by a specific viral agent regardless of how many other factors are involved in producing the cancer.

THE VIRUS OF ONE ANIMAL MAY INFECT ANOTHER SPECIES

Tumor viruses have now been proven to cross species lines to induce tumors. Some of this work was done early in cancer research using marmosets and hamsters. The greater the infectious dose of both the "helper" and primary virus, the higher is the occurrence of induced cancer. Human leukemia was transmitted to Syrian hamsters in 1967 by Dr. Sidney Farber of the Children's Cancer Research Foundation in Boston. (104) Herpes simplex type II from a human genital lesion was used by Doctors Ronald Duff and Fred Rapp of the Milton Hershey Medical Center of Pennsylvania State in making animal cells cancerous. The resulting transformed cells subsequently produced malignant tumors when injected into newborn hamsters. (105) Viral particles have been discovered in "normal" dogs living in direct contact with leukemic children. Additional confirmation of cross of species lines by cancer viruses has been obtained from the Rous sarcoma virus transmission to rabbits, dogs, mice, and hamsters. (106) (See Appendix C)

For many years, the household cat has been suspected of transmitting leukemia to humans. (107) Cat lymphoma is believed by some investigators to be transmitted from cat to cat, (108) but the question arises, can the cat leukemia and lymphoma virus cause cancer in man? Several reports have confidently declared no association between animals and human leukemia, but most of these reports were prior to 1973. (109) An epidemiologic study in 1973 revealed evidence that linked cases of human leukemia to contact with pets. Investigation focused largely on pet illnesses or death occurring in the year before the diagnosis of leukemia; and in regard to childhood cases, pet deaths that had occurred since the child's birth. The association between human leukemia and cats is stronger for ill cats, and is significant also for birds and dogs. The relative risk increases with the age of the pet. (110)

Children, ages one to fourteen, have roughly double the risk of leukemia if they have been exposed at any time during their lives to a sick cat or one which died. This finding has now been confirmed in approximately 1,400 cases. Other animals, including ill or dead canaries, parakeets, and pet dogs, show less risk of human leukemia association than cats. (111)

Malignant lymphoma is the most common cancer in cats. The causative virus can be grown in human cells in a test tube. Pregnant mothers or young children in contact with cats may be far more susceptible than others in the population. This may be an important manner in which humans, especially children, obtain leukemia or lymphoma. Leukemic cats should not be cared for in their owner's homes.

Dog, cat, and pig lymphomas have been shown to be of the same histologic type as human Burkitt's lymphoma. Lymphomas are not uncommon in these animals, particularly dogs. We should weight heavily the evidence that identical structural features between animal and human cancers reflect a common agent. (112)

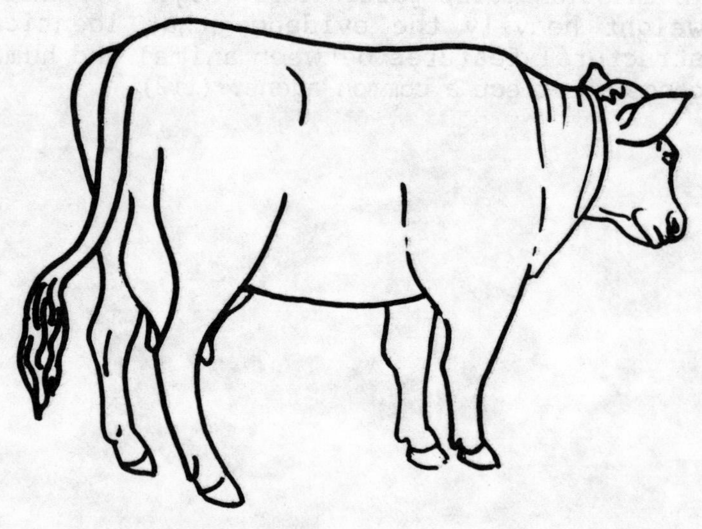

CHAPTER FIVE
The Extent of Cancer

LEUKEMIA AND LYMPHOMA

During the past forty years, the incidence of some cancers has increased by as much as 200%. The increasing death rate is typified by the unrelenting advance year by year in Georgia from 100.9 cases per 100,000 in 1960 to 131.0 in 1971. There has been a corresponding increase in malignant lymphoma and leukemia of cattle in America and Europe in recent years. Dr. Henry Lemon of of the University of Nebraska Cancer Research Institute sees a link between human leukemia and cattle leukemia. "Histologically, the blood cancer in cattle resembles lymphosarcoma and leukemia (in humans) to a 'T'." Dr. Lemon notes that dairy-rich Denmark has a leulemia incidence double that of any other western European nation, and a high rate of cattle leukosis. The Danes now have a national program to kill off leukotic cattle. A history of milk drinking has been a prominent feature in patients with leukemia states Dr. Lemon. (113) Cancer incidence throughout the world bears a direct relationship in the countries having big dairy industries.

Cattle and dairy farmers show an excess of deaths due to leukemia over a matched control group, selected from the general population. Poultry farmers are also linked with greater frequencies of leukemia. This finding is all the more striking since other rural residents consistently reveal that the total cancer mortality is much lower among them than among urban citizens. It seems logical "to relate this excess (mortality) to the known predisposition of chickens to mortality from Marek's disease," (fowl leukosis) says Dr. Samuel Milham, Jr., an epidemiologist at Washington State Division of Health in Olympia. (114)

Forty thousand Americans will develop leukemia and lymphoma this year, and thirty thousand of these victims will die. Leukemia accounts for about half of all cancer deaths in children between three and fifteen, and is much higher among milk-drinking children.

FACTORS WHICH INCREASE SUSCEPTIBILITY TO CANCER

Ammonia increases susceptibility to virus infections. One of the waste products of protein digestion is ammonia, a substance harmful to man and animals. Americans may be increasing their incidence of intestinal cancer by eating large amounts of milk, meat, eggs, and cheese. Ammonia is declared capable of changing the character of ribonucleic acid, altering the rate that thymidine is used to form deoxyribonucleic acid in living cells, and of destroying cells, thus increasing cell turnover and the opportunity cells have of becoming cancerous. All of the phenomena are stated to occur at ammonia concentrations below those usually found in man's intestine, which are high enough in the large intestine of non-vegetarians to cause severe changes in character and biochemistry of cells. (115)

Cancer-producing viruses lie dormant for a long time before they are activated by external factors (radiant energy, metabolic or hormonal factors, irritation, deficiencies in the immune system, chemicals in the blood, or environment, etc.). It is felt by many investigators that when radiation causes leukemia, it is by activation of a latent leukemia virus! There are doubtless other factors as well, such as the inevitable weakening of tissues by radiation, and the presence of altered stimuli to cell-growth--ammonia as an example.

NUTRITIONAL FACTORS

Certain nutritional factors are intimately related to the type of cancer one develops. Habitually drinking hot drinks increases one's chances of having cancer of the stomach, according to studies done in Japan. In areas where stomach cancer is high, the diet often consists of a large proportion of refined starch foods such as polished rice, white bread, and mashed potatoes; and a small proportion of fresh fruits and vegetables. Polyps and cancers of the colon are common in areas of the world where the diet contains little fiber. In trout, bears, and other animals, liver cancer has been associated with aflatoxin fed in the form of moldy foods. Aspergillus flavus is the offending mold producing the aflatoxin. Improperly stored peanuts and bread are often contaminated.

There is a correlation in man between meat consumption (or animal protein which would also include dairy products and eggs) and the incidence of cancer of the colon. There is a similar correlation with animal protein and the incidence of cancer of the breast. (116) Two hundred twenty cancer patients were compared with the same number of controls turned out to have much less fondness than the controls for raw vegetables, including lettuce, tomatoes, carrots, cole slaw, and red cabbage. Raw vegetables contain generous amounts of vitamins C and E, (117) both antioxidants acting in the body to reduce aging factors. Those who do not take generous quantities of vegetables could be expected to age at an accelerated rate and have conditions set in their cells that would encourage the development of cancer.

A high birth weight is associated with increased risk of leukemia mortality in children. (118) For several decades we have known that babies weighing over eight pounds at birth were more susceptible to diabetes (along with their mothers) than were babies weighing less than eight pounds. Since conditions which lead to diabetes also tend to lead to cancer, and since environmental factors are strongly associated with the development of both diabetes and cancer, a fruitful area to probe in prevention of cancer is the lifestyle that leads to diabetes.

OVEREATING AS A FACTOR

Abnormally high amounts of nutrients have been found to accumulate in the cells of cancerous tissue. (119) Cells may "learn" to gorge themselves with nutrients because of the custom of the person to overeat. "Why should a man need tons of meat and other high-protein foods during his lifetime when the food only breaks down into a complex of chemicals anyway before it can be used by his body?..." Large portions of unchanged proteins are taken up directly by human cells growing in culture. (120) These foreign proteins may introduce toxic by-products into the cells. Cell cultures grow at a very different rate, depending on whether they are fed whole protein or the component amino acids. With simple amino acids the cells divide only once; with the whole proteins they divide up to three times. Using more simple proteins and amino acids may exert a protective effect against excessive cell growth that might lead to cancer. Whole blood serum used as a nutrient for cells in culture brings an even greater growth--four divisions. (121) Some factor in unchanged proteins and whole serum stimulates cell division, a feature seen also in cancerous tissues.

At the University of Puerto Rico School of Medicine, a study involved sixteen mice fed hard boiled eggs and sixteen controls given regular laboratory chow. Both groups were of a cancer-prone strain. Of the controls, only two developed cancer. Of the egg-fed mice, twelve developed cancer. (122, 123) Studies show repeatedly that animal protein feeding is associated with cancer production in animals.

Leukemia in chickens accounts for annual losses to the United States poultry industry estimated in hundreds of millions of dollars.

The virus is passed from mother to chick through the egg, or from one chick to another through saliva and droppings. Some infected chickens may transmit the disease without themselves developing it. This is called latent disease and has important implications in studies of human leukemias and lymphomas. Dr. Olive Davis of Purdue University School of Veterinary Medicine developed cancer in her own lymphatic system after twenty years of working with the virus causing Marek's disease. Tumor cells from her own tumors were identical to the chicken tumor cells. (124)

Susceptibility to the development of leukosis depends on the genetic constitution, the age of exposure, horizontal infection, and the level of antibodies passed on to the chick via the egg. The earlier in life the exposure to the leukosis virus, the more likely the disease will develop. Sanitation of the living quarters and isolation of each hatch group can assist in control of the egg-borne and horizontal infections. All currently available strains of chickens are infected with the leukosis viral complex, (125) (Marek's disease) "and all chicken houses are contaminated with it.... The houses serve as reservoirs for infections of future flocks," said Dr. Ben Burmester, the developer of a vaccine against Marek's disease. (126) The chicken can still be infected by Marek's virus, but will not produce a tumor growth. The virus is a member of the herpes group of DNA viruses.

"We have discovered that the causative agent of lymphomatosis may be transmitted through eggs, coming from "carrier" hens which are healthy and in laying condition and which have not shown clinical or gross manifestations of the disease." (127) In a private communication, August, 1972, from Dr. Alexander Jackson, a researcher for about twenty years on chickens, eggs, and Rous chicken sarcoma, a statement was made that it is likely that chickens transmit human cancer, since the Rous chicken sarcoma virus has been shown to affect other animals including primates. He stated that in their home, at that time they boiled eggs for ten minutes, and baked chickens a long time rather than frying them. He believed that a sort of spore form of the cancer organism resisted ordinary cooking.

Ordinary cooking of eggs, including boiling, frying, coddling and baking, often fails to kill bacteria such as Salmonella in eggs. Many viruses are much more resistant to heat killing and drying.

LIFESTYLE FACTORS

There is an overwhelming likelihood that the lifestyle, water drinking habits, diet, previous diseases and operations, and a number of other factors unite to increase the susceptibility to cancer viruses. Considerable evidence is mounting that development of malignancies depends on the quantitative dose of virus administered (the more eggs eaten, the more virus obtained.)

A low protein diet has been shown to be beneficial in the treatment of children with leukemia (128) and as has been stated previosly, to prevent cancer development in animals. Most meats, both fresh and preserved, are in the major class of foods associated with a high bowel cancer risk. (129)

The removal of tonsils takes away a protective barrier against Hodgkin's disease. (130) Deficiencies in the immune system have been implicated in the occurrence of malignancies. (131) If the body is forced to produce large numbers of monocytes (a type of white blood cell) over long periods of time as in chronic infections, a blood cancer may eventually result. (132) Dehydration of cells may trigger cancer. (133) As one gets older body cells tend to become more dehydrated. This feature of aging is undoubtedly a factor in causing some cancers. Exercise can slow the growth of tumors. (134) These various facts serve to emphasize the desirability of following all known health laws, not just eliminating certain foods from the dietary.

There are many substances which are known to suppress various aspects of the cancer producing process in the body. For example, vitamin C as it occurs naturally inhibits the formation of nitrosamine from nitrites and amines. Flavonoids inhibit various procarcinogens, and vitamin E and sulfhydryl compounds inactivate many derived substances from procarcinogens and block certain steps in cancer production, as do vitamin A and its related retinoic acid derivatives. (135)

Breslow and Enstrom recommend several health habits to reduce cancer mortality:

1. Never smoke cigarettes
2. Take regular physical exercise
3. Drink little or no alcohol
4. Sleep 7 to 8 hours daily
5. Maintain a proper weight
6. Eat breakfast
7. Do not eat between meals

Those who persistently practice these habits were found in their study to be much less likely to die of cancer than those who practice none or only two or three. (136)

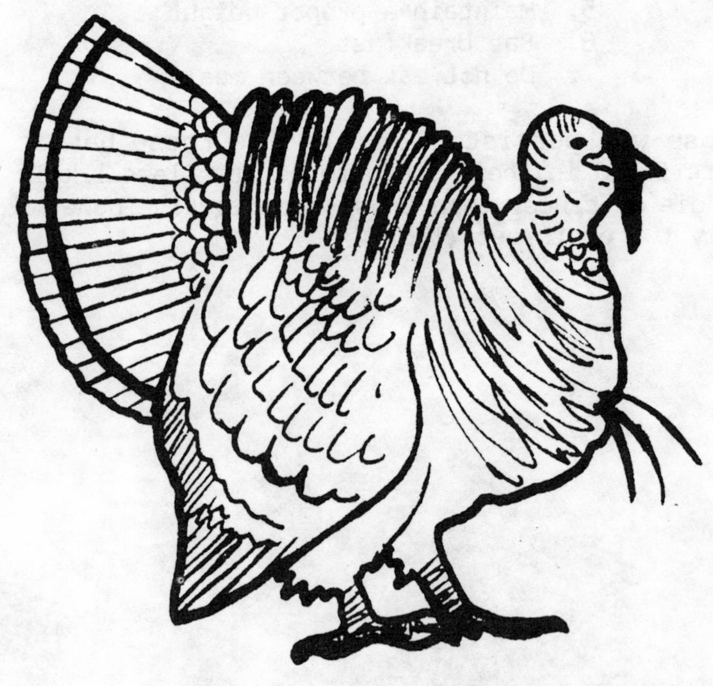

CHAPTER SIX
Foods to Use Instead of Milk and Eggs

SIMPLE AND EASY

It is not only possible but simple and easy to substitute for dairy milk and eggs in the diet. Protein, calcium, and riboflavin are generally considered the problem nutrients to replace when milk is omitted from the diet. A mixture of soy and sesame protein has a high nutritive value, comparable to milk proteins. "The cheapest way to eat twenty grams of protein is to cook up a cup of dried beans or eat four-and-a-half tablespoons of peanut butter." (137) Two pounds of soy flour contain as much protein as six dozen eggs or fifteen quarts of milk. The proteins of legumes and leafy vegetables supplement remarkably well those of cereals, and have been determined to be as efficient as proteins of animal origin. In areas where nutritional deficiency is prevalent, there is a gross shortage of good quality food of all kinds, rather than a selective shortage of animal products, the diet consisting largely of refined cornmeal, cassava root, tapioca, or white rice with practically no leafy vegetables, legumes, fruits, milk or eggs. All foods, except refined foods, contain all of the essential amino acids. From these, the body synthesizes the various amino acids it needs and forms its own proteins. (138)

KNOW YOUR NEEDS

Good milk substitutes can be obtained by a variety of combinations of sesame and sunflower seed, soy beans, and all common greens, (turnip greens, mustard, asparagus, broccoli, kale, etc.). One cup of turnip greens contains approximately the same amount of calcium as one cup of milk.

A combination of barley, whole wheat, and soy beans can be used to help replace milk in one and two year old children. It is inadvisable to take vitamin supplements, calcium, or any other purified nutrient when the diet is adequate. Split peas, lentils, or other legumes, nuts, common greens, and olives prepared in a variety of ways help take the place of milk and eggs, both from the standpoint of enjoyment and nutritional advantages.

It has long been assumed, due to the development of commercial interests of the dairy industry, that milk introduced into a a human dietary would correct any nutritional problem. Striking evidences of the error of this premise have come to the fore in such studies as those introducing milk to populations suffering from kwashiorkor or marasmus. If milk is given with an already existing vitamin A deficiency, a number of harmful effects can be expected, some of which may end up in partial or total blindness.

KEEP IT BALANCED

In Northeast Brazil, in a population having a serious deficiency of vitamin A, powdered milk was confidently introduced to alleviate the starvation. Immediately after the introduction of this food, young individuals began experiencing a growth spurt which further depleted the scanty stores of vitamin A from the liver. As a result, there were outbreaks of night blindness, xerophthalmia (drying of the conjunctiva and certain glands of the eye), keratomalacia (softening of the cornea), and irreversible blindness. There are balances of nutrients in the body that maintain an ideal relationship. Complex nutrient interactions occur in the body that are not only usual, but are the rule. (139) It may be better in some instances to have a total nutritional deficit than to have nutritional deficits in specific areas and surpluses in others.

If one suspects his diet to be deficient or inferior, a single kind of food, such as milk; or the addition of some kind of food supplements, will seldom rectify a poor diet. It is still easy to supply a balanced diet from fruits, vegetables, nuts, and whole grains in most countries. No amount of milk drinking will compensate for poor menu planning, and serious problems can result from this type of imbalance. An ideal diet consists of fruits and whole grains for breakfast, and vegetables and whole grains for lunch, all other foods being taken sparingly. Supper, if eaten, should be early, light, and composed of fruits or grains.

OSTEOPOROSIS

Even physicians will suggest that a "balanced diet" will include as much as three glasses of milk daily. It is taught, sometimes even by physicians, that to receive less calcium than the quantity supplied by three glasses of milk is dangerous. Yet, it is readily demonstrated that osteoporosis, a condition of too little mineral in the bones, results from such conditions as alcoholism, lack of exercise, and a diet containing **too many** animal products with its acidifying effect on the blood, bone and soft tissues. Unfortunately the use of 1,200 milligrams of calcium daily is prescribed for some conditions. Such a level of calcium intake endangers several systems of the body, particularly the kidneys, blood vessels, eye, skin, gallbladder, and other glandular tissues.

Many doctors are now beginning to criticize milk. It is well-known by dietitians that milk is not essential to health. Yet, some persons have a violent emotional reaction to suggestions that they stop drinking milk. Such individuals may actually suffer fatigue or other physical discomfort when milk is withdrawn from the diet. (140) It is likely that such persons are actually sensitive to milk and that milk injures their bodies. Any substance causing cellular injury can cause a true addiction. It may be that persons having an emotional attachment to milk actually suffer from a true addiction to milk.

NATIVE DIET OF JAPAN

Japan to the present day has very few domestic animals. The classic native diet of the last century was rice, seaweed, melons, and other vegetables, a variety of fruits, and fish. Generally, little or no wine or beer, milk or cheese were taken, and very little egg or meat. In fact, many people lived their lives rarely or never having eaten food of animal origin. Yet, there was (and still is) in Japan a total absence of rickets, the skeletal disease producing knock knees, bow legs and pigeon breast. There was a very low death rate in childbirth and generally easy labors. One writer commenting on this matter stated, "Now I think I am not wrong in affirming that the chief and central source of these great sanitary blessings is the absence of cow's milk." (141) Tuberculosis was also notably low, as was syphilis.

The National Dairy Council is very concerned about the trend toward strict vegetarianism and states that diets not containing animal products "pose potential hazards to one's nutrition status and general health, particularly for infants and young children." (142) In view of the large multitude of the world's poor and hungry, the National Dairy Council makes quite an admission: "Vegetarian diets can be nutritionally adequate if carefully selected. This process requires a very good knowledge of food composition and nutrition principles. As vegetarian diets become less restrictive as to nutrient sources, probability of meeting nutritional requirements increases." (Ibid) There are today untold millions of earth's population who are working productively, living happily and reproducing prolifically who have little or no knowledge of food composition and nutrition principles, but who are strictly vegetarian in their diet: no meat, milk, eggs, or cheese.

We can expect that the future will present millions more strict vegetarians than the present, as food shortages become more real in a world becoming more and more populated. In an article called **The Nutritional Adequacy of a Vegetable Substitute for Milk,** (143) R. F. A. Dean gives examples of several children who were weaned to a strictly vegetarian diet (no animal products) from a few weeks to five months of age. The infants thrived on the diet at least up to three years. Rats were also tested by experiments with mixtures of cereals and soybean products. The rats had good growth. What is needed is experimentation that will develop menus that can be easily substituted for more expensive animal products. (144)

EAT FOR STRENGTH

Several years ago we published a cookbook presenting not only recipes but also health principles which, if followed, will assist in preparing foods that will provide all the nutrients one requires to maintain health and recover from disease. The book, **Eat for Strength,** is available in both regular and oil-free editions. We recommend that babies be totally breast-fed for the first six to eight months of life, then have well-prepared table foods introduced gradually, making certain that when grains are used they are well cooked--over an hour for mushes and porridges, which guards against food sensitivities being developed because of the immature digestive tract. When the child is weaned, it should be to table foods and not to a formula.

Composition of One Cup of Milk From Each of Three Species

	Cow	Goat	Human
Calories	160	165	163
Fat (grams)	9	10	9
Protein (grams)	9	10	2.4
Calcium (mg)	288	315	88
Iron	0.1	0.2	1.5
Vitamin A	350	390	542
Vitamin C (mg)	2.0	2.0	4.9

Notice the great differences in the last five items in the chart above. Clearly, human milk is the specific milk for baby humans.

Sugars in Various Milks

Soyalac-ready to serve	65 mgs.%	1.63 gm./8 oz.
Soyalac-concentrate	112 mgs.%	2.86 gm./8 oz.
Whole dairy milk	144 mgs.%	3.67 gm./8 oz.
Breast milk	235 mgs.%	5.99 gm./8 oz.
Soyagen	63 mgs.%	1.61 gm./8 oz.
Soyamel	278 mgs.%	7.15 gm./8 oz.
Prosobee	79 mgs.%	2.03 gm./8 oz.

The National Dairy Council states that "few other foods besides dairy products contain significant amounts of biologically available calcium," (145) yet many strict vegetarians rear their children with no dairy milk. Amazingly, their dental caries are usually non-existent and broken bones are a rarity, even vanishingly rare; rickets is unheard of and may never occur except in some dark-skinned individuals who become shut up in smoggy cities away from sunshine. Tooth development should not be considered a feature of milk intake; quite the reverse. Dental caries can be initiated by bacteria that ferment any dietary carbohydrates, including milk. The "nursing bottle caries" include cavities from nursing a bottle of milk as well as a bottle of juice. Sugar induces cavities, especially sticky foods such as caramel candy, marshmallows, and other chewy candies. (146)

The relationship of calcium to phosphorus is of greater importance than the absolute quantity of calcium present in the dietary. The ideal ratio of calcium to phosphorus in the diet is approximately 1:1, except that the infant ratio should be about 1.5:1 up to six months of age, 1.35:1 up to one year of age, and then 1:1 beyond age one. (147) Foods such as processed cheese, processed meats, fabricated potato chips, refrigerator fruit turnovers, and carbonated beverages are high in phosphorus. (148) Excessive phosphates are held responsible by some for the osteoporosis (bone loss) that occurs in aging.

With the disappearance of the family cow, the flock of yard chickens and ducks, and the vanishing of the smokehouse, went the dependence of the poor on milk, eggs, and pork. These were once the low cost foods available to most of the poor. The condition has reversed at the present time, so that the poor can more readily have the foods from the vegetarian groups. "The people everywhere should be taught how to cook without milk and eggs, so far as possible, and yet have their food wholesome and palatable." (149)

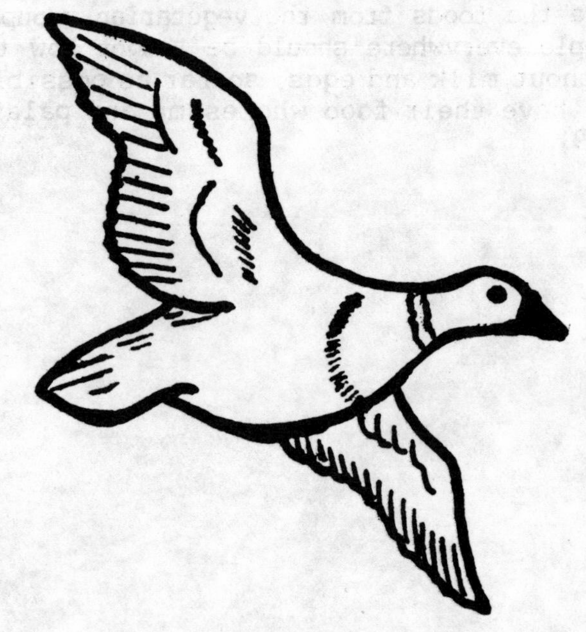

CHAPTER SEVEN
Milk-Induced Diseases

MILK INJURY, A COMMON FINDING

The emphasis given to milk drinking should be critically examined. Commercial interests have pressured people into believing they will become undernourished if they do not get milk. The fear is misplaced. Millions of healthy people never touch milk, and millions are sick because of their use of milk. Yet most of these suffering ones do not suspect milk as the culprit.

Television commercials and billboards have convinced many parents that milk is all their children need to correct an otherwise inferior diet. This is far from the case, and milk adds another feature of potential disease producing elements to the diet. Milk displaces more important foods in the diet, some of which contain nutrients essential to proper growth and development, both physical and mental. (150) Milk may cause a variety of diseases, even death. "Possible deaths related to milk hypersensitivity have received little attention. We have demonstrated that severe cardiorespiratory abnormalities can be ameliorated by withdrawal of cow's milk from the diet of the sensitive individual.

"Based on information presently available, we recommend that all children with chronic or undefined upper and lower respiratory tract disease be screened for milk precipitins, elevated serum IgE levels, and pulmonary hemosiderosis. A cause and effect relationship between symptoms and cow milk ingestion should be sought." (151)

It is difficult or impossible for the government to insure that milk or other foods of animal origin will be fit for human consumption. Unsolvable problems associated with marketing foods of animal origin range through a large number of unfortunate factors, definite fraud, illegal labeling, the addition of extenders without indicating their presence, and a potpourri of other illegal or revolting practices which cannot be controlled by any agency no matter how elaborate the enforcing body. Inflation increases the pressure to cheat.

THE MILK MYSTIQUE

There are certain customs in society which become so firmly entrenched that any examination of the tradition is considered near to sacrilege. Milk is one of these sacrosanct matters in our society, so cherished that any statement against it may be regarded with disfavor or suspicion. Furthermore, the milk advisory board and the various private industries and organizations promoting milk make certain that all nutritionists and teachers are programmed to think kindly of milk. From many directions come indications that dairy milk is not the perfect food, not even for babies. Of all mammals, man is the only one that takes milk into adult life. Dr. Frank Oski, a pediatrician from State University of New York, Upstate Medical Center in Syracuse, agrees that we must add milk to the hazardous food lists. (152)

Cliches such as "milk is the perfect food" die slowly. It is true that milk contains a wide variety of needed elements, but none of these nutrients was generated by the cow; she obtained the nutrients she put into the milk from the food she consumed: greens, legumes, and whole grains--common articles of diet. It is also true that milk contains contaminants, infectious agents, and difficult-to-handle nutrients as well. In fact, the three major nutrients of milk, butter fat, milk protein (caseine) and milk carbohydrate (lactose) are likely to cause adults to have much less than optimum health.

BY-PRODUCTS OF MILK

The milk industry has become so enormous and uses for milk so varied that many by-products of manufacturing processes are left over, and uses must be found for these substances. To prevent large losses to the milk industry, many of these products and by-products turn up in the market labeled "non-dairy," so defined by law. But those who cannot use dairy products usually cannot use these articles either.

A "filled milk" is defined as any milk, cream, or skimmed milk to which any fat or oil other than milk fat has been added. An "imitation milk" usually contains a protein such as sodium caseinate or soy protein, corn syrup solids, sugar and vegetable fat. Artificial coffee creamers are similar to imitation milks but are nutritionally inferior in regard to protein, vitamins, minerals, and sometimes fatty acid content. (153)

The milk of the species is as distinctive as the skin and hair. For baby humans, breast milk is a perfect design; for baby calves, cow's milk is perfect; but to give a baby human cow's milk is far from perfect. In fact, it may set the stage for allergies, sensitivities, and many serious sicknesses throughout life. Ellen White, a Seventh-day Adventist health educator of the last century, taught that the time would come when milk would be considered hazardous to the health. "In a short time the milk of cows will also be excluded from the diet.... In a short time it will not be safe to use anything that comes from the animal creation." (154) "There will soon be no safety in the possession of flocks or herds." (155) "...we know that the time will come when it will not be best to use milk and eggs." (156)

SUGAR AND MILK COMBINATIONS DANGEROUS

Milk taken in large quantities is undoubtedly able to encourage the development of diabetes or the hypoglycemic syndrome. Milk sugar is handled principally by the pancreas, and the large quantities of milk consumed in many parts of the United States certainly contributes to these prevalent and increasing problems. The cause of the current epidemics of diabetes mellitus probably includes smoking, lack of exercise, environmental stress, and many improper dietary habits--excessive intake of sugar and dairy products being among these. Sucrose (table sugar) and milk taken together, as is commonly done in this country, appear to be particularly dangerous. (157) That sucrose and saturated fats may potentiate each other has not been investigated at great depth, but the prevalence in the Western world of recipes that contain this combination suggests an incrimination of this combination. (158, 159) The simultaneous intake of sucrose and milk appears to make growth hormone more active. The pancreas is stimulated in its metabolic activity, resulting in an increased need for carbohydrates, the uptake of which is blocked by the free fatty acids from milk. (160) The influence of milk-sugar combinations on growth hormone may explain the rapid growth and overgrowth of children who consume a lot of sweetened milk foods.

Considering its widespread use, even to the point of force feeding, how strange that very little investigation has been done along the lines of establishing with certainty that milk satisfies all the expectations of the consumer and claims of the producer. Many problems have been identified even with the small amount of research that has been done. Milk may contribute to the formation of kidney stones, may cause intestinal malabsorption and diarrhea, and may even **cause** malnourishment of older infants, especially leading to iron deficiency anemia. (161) Good evidence has been presented that milk products are associated with the development of cancer, skin lesions, musculoskeletal abnormalities, pulmonary obstruction, immunological disorders, and liver function abnormalities. As far back as 1931, the diseases of cattle transmitted to men through milk were receiving a prominent position in medical literature. (162)

There are six categories of milk-induced diseases: those from the fat of milk, the protein, the carbohydrate, the contaminants, food intolerance, and allergies to milk. These diseases will be discussed in the next several chapters.

CHAPTER EIGHT
Diseases From Milk Fat

FAT ALTERS RED BLOOD CELLS AND CIRCULATION

Commercial cream is 40% fat, butter is 80% fat. Red blood cells can cluster together in tight wads following the ingestion of any kind of fat. Milk or butter fat, cream, and other fats are capable of causing clumping together of red blood cells inside of blood vessels. This interesting phenomenon may be seen in the hamster by examining the small blood vessels in the cheek pouch after the animal has taken cream or butter fat. Controls receiving skimmed milk or other kinds of foods do not show these changes. It has been postulated that these clusters of red blood cells could cause strokes or a reduced mentality in the elderly. (163)

Perhaps the most hazardous time after eating fats is immediately following the meal and for about one hour afterward. During this time effort should be put forth to insure a brisk circulation of blood. If the blood moves slowly there is greater encouragement of the formation of the red blood cell clusters. Furthermore, sludge of fat droplets can form in the large lymph channels in the chest and abdomen during inactivity and float to blood vessels where they cause some degree of interference with blood flow--perhaps even blockage. The best practice is to engage in some form of mild exercise just after eating to insure a brisk circulation of blood.

Many infants are born with high blood cholesterol levels. Coronary risk factors exist in childhood, and plaques of atherosclerosis in heart and arteries are formed early in life. (164) It is generally accepted that milk intake by the mother during pregnancy and after delivery, as well as that taken by the newborn greatly contributes to this problem.

An inducement to breast-feeding is that in human mother's milk there is a compound that blocks cholesterol synthesis by the liver. (165) Mexican children who use little or no milk have half the blood cholesterol levels of Wisconsin children. (166) In American children who come to autopsy from whatever cause, fatty streaks in the blood vessels may be seen in infancy and childhood with fibrous plaques being formed in the teenage years.

For a number of decades, heart and artery disease, caused by an increase of cholesterol, and other blood fats, have been recognized as being associated with milk. Pure vegetarians have significantly lower serum cholesterol levels than either lactovegetarians or non-vegetarians. (167) While most authorities are agreed that the fat in milk is a major cause of hardening of the arteries, there are investigators, growing in number, who believe a virus or some other factor from milk is primarily responsible for the hardening of the arteries seen when milk consumption is high.

AGING FATS IN CHEESE-MAKING

Aging of milk fats in the cheese-making process may hold yet another hazard to consumers. It was found by accident that injurious products develop in cholesterol upon aging. A researcher bought a large quantity of cholesterol for animal experimentation. He began to develop variable and unexpected results with the cholesterol after it had aged a number of months. A chemical analysis of the cholesterol revealed three products of degradation which could cause death of muscle fibers in artery walls. A prominent theory of atherosclerosis development holds that the initial injury is in the muscle fibers of the artery walls, not in the lining cells as formerly universally accepted. Fats subsequently deposit in the areas where the injury occurred in the muscle cells. (168)

It will not solve the problem of altered blood chemistries to use defatted milk. It was discovered in the making of dairy butter, that the phospholipids go with the buttermilk and cholesterol goes with the butter fat. When the phospholipids and cholesterol are kept together, the phospholipids tend to reduce the quantity of cholesterol that stays in the blood stream. As with all foods, the balance found naturally is ideal for its proper function in the body, illustrating the carefulness and precision of the loving Creator in every design having to do with the welfare of His creatures.

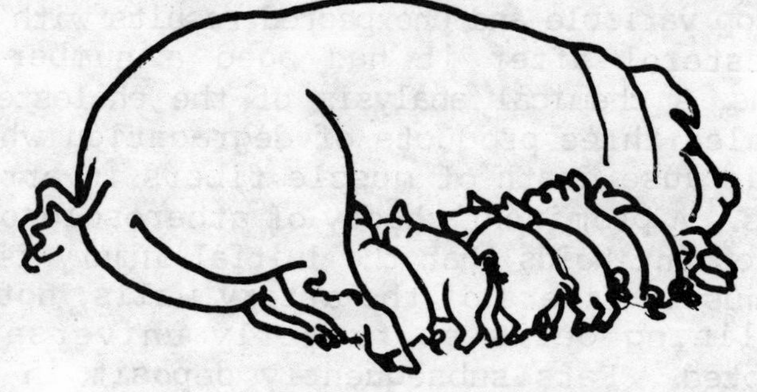

CHAPTER NINE
Proteins and Amino Acids in Milk

THE PROTEIN OF MILK

It is difficult for adults to digest milk protein. The amino acid balance of caseine, the principal protein of milk, is not ideal for adults. Babies are equipped with rennin, a special enzyme for the digestion of caseine, and adults, who lack this enzyme, often suffer from allergies to milk protein. Human milk has little caseine and much lactalbumin, while cow's milk presents the opposite picture. And, of course, lactalbumin is the best protein for human growth. Caseine is less valuable for human growth, and less easily digested, the resulting incompletely digested protein fragments being available to cause allergies. Babies who are denied mother's milk are truly in a poverty program. The word "unfair" applies to them.

Only 60% of caseine can be retained by the body. It would seem wise to deliver protein to underdeveloped areas in some other form than milk solids, the form often selected by United States officials. Legumes and grains would be more helpful. Milk protein intolerance can apparently damage the mucosa of the gastrointestinal tract and produce enzyme deficiency and mucosal damage. (170) There has been some discussion in recent years that in addition to the fat, milk protein along with other food allergens, may also promote the development of atherosclerosis. (171, 172) A high protein diet can actually be dangerous to the body, as it can increase the need for vitamin B-12, trigger loss of calcium from bone, and can actually break down some protein tissues. (173)

Heated milk protein has been postulated to be one of the causes of the sudden steep rise in coronary heart disease which began about one or two years after the widespread introduction of pasteurized milk in 1922. Milk fat correlates **less well** than milk protein with the increase in coronary heart disease. (174)

MILK CAUSES DROWSINESS

Milk drinking has been associated with mental symptoms. Warm milk at bedtime has been improperly used to induce sleep. While food at bedtime may help the person to be drowsy, the resulting sleep does not bring the refreshing rest that sleep on an empty stomach brings, and the person feels tired in the morning. Since L-tryptophane, a substance high in meat and milk, causes drowsiness and sleep as successfully as do drugs (175) those who take milk or meat late at night are likely to sleep the sleep of the drugged. Milk taken for lunch often causes afternoon drowsiness. Sleeping when milk is in the stomach is likely to cause hiatus hernia symptoms or heartburn.

LEUCINE AND BLOOD SUGAR

The use of dairy products with their high leucine content causes a profound fall in blood glucose concentration in many individuals, some having such low blood sugar levels that cerebral damage occurs. Convulsive seizures are known to be associated with a diet high in leucine, probably because of the reactive hypoglycemia induced by leucine. A case to illustrate this condition is that of a 10-month-old black female who was otherwise healthy, until she was found unconscious and taken to the hospital. A week later she had a second such episode, but this time it was observed to follow a convulsive seizure. For sixteen weeks she suffered many convulsive seizures, both in the fasting state and following meals. When milk was entirely withdrawn from her diet for three months, she had but one mild convulsive seizure. When milk was reintroduced on a trial basis, she had two seizures the first day and several more subsequently. The seizures were associated with severe low blood sugar levels, the laboratory reports were always below 50 when checked after meals containing milk. (176)

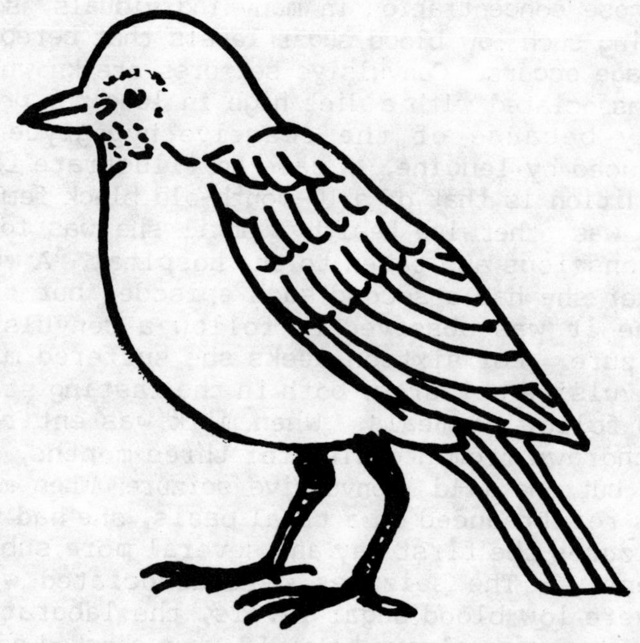

CHAPTER TEN
Vitamin-Mineral Content of Milk

MINERAL BALANCE NOT IDEAL FOR HUMANS

As a principal food, the vitamin-mineral balance of milk is not ideal for children or adults. There is too much sodium, too little vitamin C, and too little iron. Under some conditions, milk interferes with the absorption of iron. It is believed to bind zinc in a way that reduces its utilization by the body. Zinc is an important substance in the nutrition of man. Milk is low in zinc. Nuts, dry legumes, and whole grains contain up to ten times more zinc than milk. (177) Any degree of lactose intolerance can be expected to enhance the problem of low zinc content in milk.

The mineral balance of milk is not the only matter to cause concern, but the total number of waste product non-metabolizable dietary components, especially electrolytes which are spoken of as the "renal solute load" can be greatly increased by milk. Electrolytes taken in excess of the needs of the body, and the nitrogenous compounds which result from the digestion and metabolism of protein can put quite a load on the kidneys. This matter becomes especially important when there is a low appetite for water, and in infants and elderly people with a low fluid intake. This group is often being fed calorically concentrated diets, particularly if there is an abnormally high loss of water either through the kidneys, the skin, or the bowels, as in fever, elevated environmental temperature, diarrhea, or in the use of medicinal diuretics, or in cases of hyperventilation. Overconcentrated formulas for infants and children are risky, and may permanently injure the kidneys or cause death. Formulas prepared from improperly diluted evaporated milk or various powdered milk formulas or supplements that may be added represent a hazard to infants who have functionally immature kidneys. (178)

VITAMIN D AND MAGNESIUM

Vitamin D (which is added to commercial milk) in too great a quantity causes loss of magnesium from heart muscle. Some authorities believe that magnesium loss is what precipitates heart attacks. Rats fed five times the usual magnesium in the diet are protected from the heart attacks they could get from excess vitamin D. Adding potentially toxic substances such as vitamin D to milk is not wise. The American Academy of Pediatrics recommends no more than 400 units of vitamin D from all sources be consumed daily. Hardening of bones, renal calcification, and severe mental retardation in offspring have all been reported from a high vitamin D intake. (179)

MILK INCREASES THE NEED FOR MANY NUTRIENTS

Babies who have diarrhea, hair loss, weight loss, and who develop bright red lesions in the diaper area, spreading to the limbs, face, and bodily orifices may be suffering from zinc deficiency. Human milk contains a protein which assists in the absorption of zinc in newborns. (180) All kinds of nuts and seeds are relatively good sources of zinc. Dairy milk is a poor source of both zinc, (181) and iron. Further, a high calcium intake, especially in the presence of phytic acid, depresses the absorption of zinc. (182) Since milk is both a poor source of zinc and a high source of calcium, it would be wise to avoid milk and to give foods that contain a good zinc level to babies having these symptoms. (183) Since refined foods also generally contain low levels of zinc, these articles should also be avoided as a general rule.

The use of milk increases the need for vitamin A, and probably also iron, calcium, zinc, and vitamin B-12. The objective in nutrition is to obtain the most safe, reasonable, and economical foods in their most natural possible state, prepared in a simple yet tasty way, and served in a pleasant and nice manner.

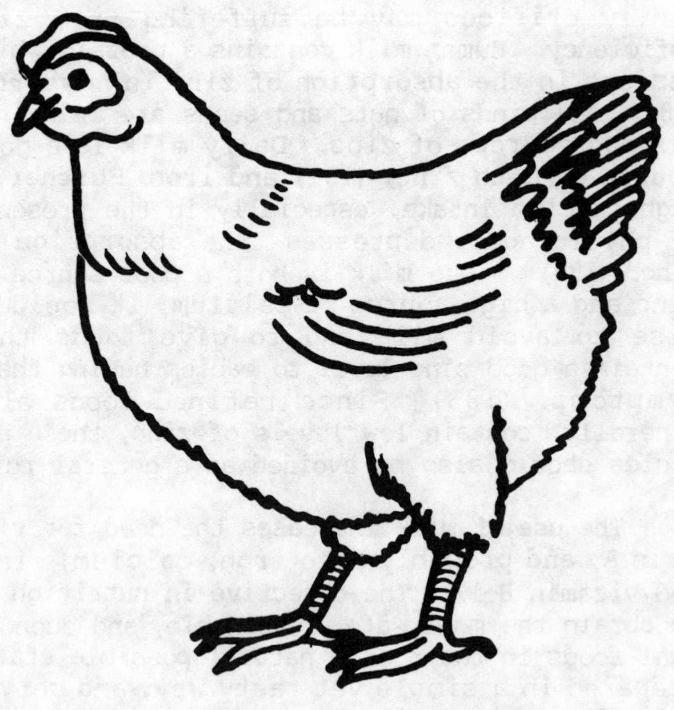

CHAPTER ELEVEN
Xanthine Oxidase — A New Culprit?

WHAT CAUSES HEART AND ARTERY DISEASE?

Dairy milk is a rich source of xanthine oxidase, an enzyme occurring naturally in milk. Goat and sheep milk contains less xanthine oxidase than cow's milk. Boiling, but not homogenization or pasteurization will destroy xanthine oxidase. (184) The natural function of xanthine oxidase is to control the last stages of purine metabolism with its end-product, uric acid, the waste product related to gout.

Folic acid is a xanthine oxidase inhibitor and prevents or arrests the progress of dietary atherosclerosis. There is a significant decline in angina and repeated heart attacks in persons treated with folic acid, (185) supporting the idea that xanthine oxidase is active in the cause of artery disease.

In heart and artery disease, xanthine oxidase may chemically produce the injury that initiates atherosclerotic lesions in the vessel walls by depleting the plasmalogen content of arterial and heart tissues. When this enzyme is biochemically unavailable, as in population groups as in France or India who do not homogenize their milk, but do boil the milk, or in societies where little or no milk is taken, coronary artery disease is extremely low. In one study of atherosclerotic persons, 73 of 94 subjects were found to have antibodies to bovine milk xanthine oxidase.

MILKSHAKES AND TONSILLECTOMY

There are highly significant correlations between heavy milkshake and milk consumption in early life, and the presence of abnormal blood fat patterns, low serum glucose levels, (hypoglycemia, which predicts a tendency toward diabetes) and the incidence of tonsillectomy at age ten or later. All of these factors in the history **also** correlate with the presence of antibodies to bovine milk xanthine oxidase. It appears that the gastrointestinal tract can learn to take up bovine milk xanthine oxidase directly without digesting it. (186) Perhaps the function of completely digesting milk is injured by overconsumption of milk in early life, and especially by the use of milk-sugar combinations such as milkshakes or sweetened cereals and milk.

Dr. Kurt A. Oster, a leading cardiologist, believes that xanthine oxidase in milk is more related to the development of atherosclerosis than are milk fats (187) and that it is the process of homogenizing milk and breaking up its fat into the tiny particles for even distribution through the milk, which enables portions of milk to be absorbed directly into the blood stream from the gastrointestinal tract. Along with these finely divided particles of fat, the xanthine oxidase goes directly through the walls of the intestines and acts chemically to injure the artery walls and heart tissues as previously mentioned. (188)

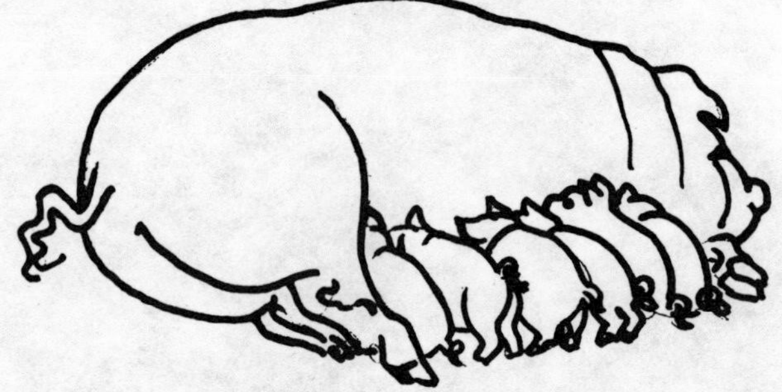

CHAPTER TWELVE
Diseases Caused by Contaminants in Milk

THINGS GET INTO MILK

Female sex hormones and thyroid hormones are administered to cows to increase milk yield. Every year, in this country, antibiotics worth 478 million dollars are added to animal feeds to increase milk yield. The antibiotics and hormones used in the feed turn up in both the milk and the meat from these animals. Antibiotic-resistant bacteria are developing as a result of repeated small exposures to the antibiotics, and are being fed continually into the population from this source. (189)

Certain toxic substances are absorbed into the blood more easily when in the presence of particular foods that act as helpers. Lead bears such a relationship to milk, being absorbed more readily in the presence of milk. (190) More lead can be absorbed by the animal if his feed contains swill (refuse food mixed with milk condemned by the inspectors). High lead levels then appear in the tissues of animals fed contaminated feed. Several years ago, there was a widely publicized case in the newspapers of a man who fed contaminated feed to his hogs. His wife and two children died from the lead-contaminated meat, and another child was permanently brain-damaged from the toxic effects on the nerves.

Cadmium is known to be associated with deaths from kidney and artery disease. Diet and drinking water are the chief sources of human cadmium intake. Milk cadmium is used as a crude index of the total dietary cadmium. It has been shown that if milk consumed in the spring has a high cadmium level, there will be a high positive correlation with deaths from heart and blood vessel disease later that year. (191)

Unwashed vegetation containing dangerous radionuclides, eaten by cattle and excreted in the milk, is found to be an important cause of man's dietary intake of environmental radioactivity. Fresh milk contains several of the biologically important radionuclides. Strontium 89, strontium 90, iodine 131, barium 140, and cesium 137 are sources of environmental radioactivity, all of which occur in milk. (192) Strontium 90, closely resembling calcium in its chemical behavior, follows the food chain in the same way that calcium does from the soil, into grass, into milk, and finally into children, being lodged in the growing bones of children. Embedded in bone it exposes nearby cells to beta radiation, increasing the lifetime risk of cancer.

GOAT'S MILK NOT THE ANSWER

The levels of strontium 90 in the milk produced nearby, and in the diet of those living near Connecticut nuclear power plants were greater when checked in 1976 than in areas far removed from nuclear power plants. (193) Nor is taking goat's milk the answer, as goat's milk was found to be higher in strontium 90 than cow's milk.

Scientists investigating the case of a baby born with severe bone deformities of his arms and legs learned that his mother had used goat's milk during pregnancy. The goat had given birth to kids with similar deformities, and a dog, also given goat's milk had given birth to deformed pups. The researchers felt that a toxic forage plant eaten by the goat produced the deformities. (248)

Pesticides such as DDT, appear in milk samples, as do polychlorinated biphenyls (PCBs). (194) The amounts found exceed the Food and Drug Administration maximums. PCBs are concentrated in milk fat, and their behavior is quite similar to chlorinated hydrocarbon residues. (195) The danger from milk was recently underscored because of the contamination of milk by PBBs (polybrominated biphenyls). Thousands of people in Michigan in 1973 were exposed to these substances before the contamination was discovered. (196)

Female sex hormones and other hormone substances are often administered to cattle. In cows, the volume of milk produced is increased by 30 percent (with a corresponding increase in milk solids) by giving thyroxin or thyroglobulin.

When cattle eat bracken fern, toxic substances from the fern appear in the milk. Such milk has been found to contain certain fractions demonstrated to cause mutagenic activity in cells, increasing the risk of deformities in babies and cancer in all ages. (197) Aflatoxin, the potent cancer-producing agent produced by fungi, has been discovered in significant quantities in milk. It gets into milk from the growth of fungi in the feed of the animal. (198)

GOITERS IN TASMANIA

A goitrogenic substance was found in milk as early as 1957. (199) It is believed by some that the calcium of milk may act as a goitrogen. (200) It has also been suggested that since cattle consume large quantities of the plant genus Brassica which includes cabbages, mustards, rapes, kale and turnips, in their forage material, and are fed whole peanuts, that goitrogens become concentrated in milk from this source. (201)

In Tasmania, an epidemic of goiters occurred in school children. It was observed that children who drank milk developed the goiters, and those who did not drink milk had no goiters. On investigation, it was discovered that the local cattle had been fed fodder made from cabbages and related greens. These greens contain a goitrogenic agent, thiourea. (202) The thiourea is excreted in the milk. It was this substance which gave the school children goiter.

CHAPTER THIRTEEN
Food Intolerance From Milk

A WIDESPREAD CONDITION

Food intolerance is any unwanted reaction from food and includes food allergies. Definite allergies to milk will be considered separately. A food intolerance to milk is caused by inability to absorb, digest, or handle the chemical components in milk. It can be caused by a chemical incompatibility between various parts of the milk and human chemicals.

RECTAL BLEEDING

One type of such disease in humans is that of rectal bleeding due to milk. A 38-year-old woman with a persistent seven year history of rectal bleeding stopped drinking milk and her rectal bleeding stopped. When she was challenged with a test dose of milk on several occasions, her rectal bleeding promptly returned. (203)

ULCERATIVE COLITIS

Milk has been associated with ulcerative colitis at least since 1926. One 12-year-old girl had the disease approximately two years, and cleared entirely after stopping the use of milk. Her symptoms would become painfully evident by even the occasional use of a small quantity of milk.

Our experience with many patients with ulcerative colitis supports the findings of other physicians that ulcerative colitis patients get along much better, and many have hope of complete cure if the diet is carefully controlled. Milk is number one on the list of foods which may cause trouble for persons with ulcerative colitis. Dr. I. Dodd Wilson believes that a reasonable approach to patients having acute attacks of ulcerative colitis might be to ban milk. (204) We have given a diet free from all dairy products to our ulcerative colitis patients for years, and find that their remissions are longer, relapses are fewer (205) and some are entirely cured.

PEPTIC ULCER TREATMENT?

A 57-year-old man with peptic ulcer was placed on a diet consisting of milk and cream every hour on the half-hour and one gram of calcium carbonate every hour on the hour with 2.5 grams of magnesium oxide daily. After three weeks he became drowsy, vomited, and had epigastric pain. Blood chemistry determination showed abnormal blood urea, creatinine, calcium (16 mgs. %), phosphorus and carbon dioxide. It was found that he had been eating from one-fourth to one-half pound of cheese daily, which contains the amount of nutrients equivalent to that contained in from one pint to one quart of milk daily. He was found to have renal damage, which apparently returned to normal after his treatment routine was changed. (206)

MANY CHILDHOOD DISORDERS CAN BE MILK SENSITIVITIES

Among the childhood disorders associated with milk drinking are loss of appetite, anemia, fretfulness, bedwetting, constipation, bloating, abdominal pains, and diarrhea. (207, 208)

Bedwetting can often be successfully treated by putting the child on a diet free from milk. In one study, 100 children with bedwetting were placed on a diet containing no milk. At least half of the children stopped bedwetting with the change in diet. Of the others, forty responded partially, but the remaining ten apparently did not respond to the milk-free diet. In Chapter Ten the subject of the nerve depressing influence of certain amino acids of milk is discussed. It may be through this mechanism that milk causes bedwetting. It is speculated that milk may lower a child's voiding reflex threshold because of an inhibition of certain centers in the brain stem, resulting in involuntary voiding. (209)

Because of the influence of milk or milk sensitivity on the central nervous system, a milk sensitivity or intolerance can present a number of symptoms of irritation of the nervous system in children, such as learning disability, headache, and just plain feeling bad. Cases have been described in all these categories. Multiple sclerosis is related to milk production and consumption in a way not fully understood. Some investigators believe drinking milk during the period of most rapid brain development, and past the normal weaning age is detrimental, and that studies should be directed toward investigating the role of milk, or some infectious or toxic agent contained in milk, in causing multiple sclerosis. (210)

COLIC, COLDS, AND CHILDHOOD HYPERTENSION

Dairy milk has been associated with infantile colic, even in breast-fed infants; the mother drinks the milk and the baby develops infantile colic. When the mother is put on a diet free of dairy milk protein, the colic disappears promptly. If the mother starts drinking milk again, as many as twelve out of thirteen cases of infantile colic in breast-fed infants can be expected to reappear. If an infant who has shown infantile colic through the mother's milk drinking is challenged directly with the milk, four out of five will usually react promptly by developing a bout of colic. The treatment of colic in breast-fed infants should begin by removing milk from the diet of the mother. (211)

When a child has repeated "colds," or other respiratory diseases, the mother should always think of milk allergy. A small Canadian boy having his eighth attack of pneumonia at twelve months of age was merely taken off milk and dairy products; he recovered and had no subsequent attacks. Many children who suffer repeatedly from bronchitis and pneumonia turn out to have milk allergies or sensitivities to other common foods (citrus fruits, juices, eggs, pork, coffee, tea, colas, chocolate, artificial coloring and flavoring agents, spices, cane sugar, tomatoes, strawberries, breads and cereals, etc. (212, 213, 214)

Childhood hypertension is associated with a high intake of sodium and a high intake of calories. By restricting both salt and calorie intake, any predisposition that a child may have to develop hypertension can be controlled. Reducing salt intake to small amounts in diets of persons with high blood pressure almost always produces a favorable blood pressure response. In some individuals, however, it is necessary to eliminate entirely both salt and oil. It is certainly prudent to avoid heavy salting and the large intake of high fat foods common among children. Since milk naturally possesses a high sodium content and is a high calorie food, its use in childhood hypertension is contraindicated. (215) Ideally children should not even become acquainted with milkshakes, commercial candies and ice cream, fried snack foods and other concentrated and calorically dense foods.

The presence of digested blood in the stools (stools have a black, tarry color) has been described in children as a result of milk drinking. A 19-month-old infant whose stools were "pitch black" had anemia with a hemoglobin of eight grams, which completely cleared on withdrawing milk. (216) Any child with chronic diarrhea, bloody, or black stools, an increase in the number of eosinophils in the blood, eczema, hives, asthma, or other signs of allergy should be investigated for milk intolerance. If the symptoms continue when switching to soy milk, the diagnosis is still not ruled out, as at least 20% of patients intolerant to milk are also intolerant to soy protein. (217) Weight loss, vomiting, and diarrhea, associated with chemical abnormalities in the blood are also found with soy protein intolerance. (218)

Infancy and childhood is the time when exposure to milk is most common. Infancy and childhood are also the periods in life when the immune mechanism is as yet underdeveloped. Protection of children from infections may need to include protection from milk. Caseine, the principal protein in milk is especially likely to injure the lining of the first portion of the small bowel in young infants who have acute infectious enteritis. It is recognized that babies recovering from enteritis should not be given a diet containing milk or foods containing lactose (milk sugar) or caseine (milk protein). (219)

INFANTILE DIARRHEA

It is quite likely that infantile diarrhea is transmitted to babies through dairy products. Outbreaks of diarrhea in children often follow the geographical area served by a single dairy. When calves at the dairy are suffering an epidemic of diarrhea, it is not uncommon to have an epidemic of infantile diarrhea among the babies in the corresponding community at the same time. This indicates that both outbreaks are due to the same virus. Infantile diarrhea is sometimes life-threatening for a baby. With the production of fifteen to twenty watery stools within a few hours, the infant becomes dangerously dehydrated. To prevent diarrhea in infants, usually the only thing needed is to insure breast-feeding, and another serious disease of babies is eliminated.

I well remember the case of a friendly, good-natured, black nurse who worked in the pediatrics department during my internship. She had had her first child after twelve years of marriage. Shortly after the birth of the baby, it was discovered that the mother had a urinary tract malformation, and must never have another pregnancy. This premium baby was the mother's pride and joy. Unfortunate circumstances forced her to return to work when the baby was nearly three months old. She reluctantly put the baby on formula and left the baby with the grandmother during her work shift. One day the baby became sick with diarrhea and fever. That night, the baby had several stools during a short time, and became moribund before morning. She rushed the baby to the hospital, burst into the pediatrics emergency room with the unconscious baby in her arms. I worked with the pediatrics staff over the baby for several anxious hours before it died. The poor mother was inconsolable. The distressed mourning of that mother is a painful memory which constantly encourages me to educate all mothers everywhere to breast-feed their babies. Many milk-borne infections that might snuff out the life of some infant, or cause much suffering and grief, may be avoided thereby.

FEEDING PROBLEMS

A child may develop a chronic feeding problem because of too much milk, with an aversion to breakfast, a preference for soft carbohydrate foods that require little chewing. The child may develop a problem with constipation, and may seem always to have a cold. He may be overweight or underweight. The parents may be anxious about his getting "enough milk" which they have been educated to believe is "nature's most nearly perfect food." He is often a poor sleeper. (220)

Milk is a common cause of constipation, or of alternating diarrhea and constipation. To get rid of constipation, milk should be eliminated, and fruits, vegetables, and whole grains should be added in generous quantities to the diet. Many times if such an individual adds even a small amount of milk the constipation returns immediately. (221) This person may be tempted to believe that a small quantity of milk could not possibly be instrumental in bringing on his constipation, but faithful attention to total elimination of milk from the diet will often be very rewarding.

CHAPTER FOURTEEN
Lactose

LACTOSE SENSITIVITY—A LARGE PROBLEM

Lactose (milk sugar) is the principal carbohydrate of milk, and often causes symptoms ranging from mild to serious, mainly gastrointestinal, in a large percentage of persons who use dairy products. When a patient has vague gastrointestinal complaints, it is always necesary to think of lactose intolerance. Lactase is an enzyme that helps in the digestion of lactose, and if there is incomplete digestion of milk, irritation can result, or the formation of gas or acids. Thirty-three million Americans have low lactase levels. There is a normal, post-weaning reduction in lactase activity in all mammals. If lactose cannot be digested because of insufficient lactase, the unsplit lactose passes into the colon where fermentation produces gas, alcohols, and irritating organic acids such as lactic and acetic acids. There is a great likelihood that intestinal production of the enzyme lactase is absent or low in persons with digestive complaints at all ages. An acid stool with a pH of less than six is significant in making the diagnosis of lactase insufficiency. (222)

OFTEN MISDIAGNOSED

Many persons with misdiagnosed lactose intolerance have been said to have functional bowel disease, nervous or ulcerative colitis, spastic, neurotic, or irritable bowel syndrome. These persons suffer from diarrhea, nausea, decramps, vomiting and abdominal pain. Some degree of lactose intolerance is present in almost 100% of adult Africans, Orientals, and American Indians, and 60 to 70% of descendants of Ashkenazi Jews, black Americans, and Mexican-Americans. Ten to fifteen percent of white Americans of Scandinavian or Northern European descent are lactose intolerant. Forty percent of United States black elementary students and 75% of black teen-agers are intolerant to milk. Approximately 80% of the world's population does not produce sufficient lactase, and consequently cannot completely split the lactose present in any reasonable serving of dairy products. In these low lactase producers, symptoms are common. Most infants with demonstrated lactose intolerance will have a complete relief of abdominal pain upon withdrawing milk and milk products from the diet. (223)

In many parts of China, the use of milk and eggs is thought of with disgust and aversion, much as Americans regard with disgust the use of blood as food or beverage. Many Chinese develop abdominal discomfort after drinking milk due to an inability to metabolize lactose. Lactose intolerance producing aversion to milk may be one physiological mechanism in the development of culturally determined attitudes toward food. (224) An easy way to make the diagnosis of lactose intolerance is by stopping the milk intake for about a week, then giving two glasses of cold milk (which produces symptoms more readily than warm milk). It can thereby be easily determined if there is a relationship between milk drinking and the physical complaints. (225)

MILK DISTRIBUTION PROGRAMS—WHO BENEFITS?

The mandatory milk distribution programs in school lunchrooms are not only not beneficial, but are probably harmful to most non-Caucasians. (226) Elevated temperatures, vomiting, or diarrhea with weight loss are signs of lactose sensitivity, along with a multiplicity of other symptoms related to the abdomen or to other systems. (227) Lactase deficiency may lead to the development of cataracts since the improper digestion of milk can allow certain parts of the milk, notably galactose, to accumulate, and cataracts are more common when galactose is high in the diet.

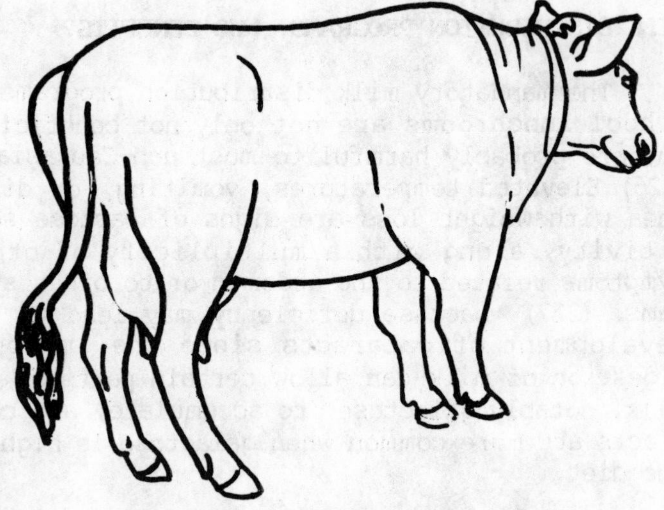

CHAPTER FIFTEEN
Allergies to Dairy Products

BEGIN AT BIRTH TO PREVENT ALLERGIES

The tendency to develop allergies begins early in life. If we wish to avoid a lifetime battle with allergies, we must begin at least at birth with breast-feeding. Human milk contains up to six times as much vitamin E as does cow's milk, and about twice as much selenium, according to Dr. Donald Money of Wallaceville Animal Research Center in New Zealand.

Antibodies are substances produced by the body in response to the stimulus of an irritating foreign substance (antigen). Since antibodies are proteins of the globulin fraction, antibodies are called "immune globulins," shortened to Ig. Deficiencies and surpluses of the immune globulins (antibodies) are related to allergies.

Immune globulins are capable of serving many functions, only one of which is combating invading germs after they obtain entry to the body. One immune globulin, IgA, is excreted in intestinal mucus, and is thought to provide powerful local protection against infection, particularly viral. A high incidence of antibodies to milk proteins has been recorded in patients deficient in IgA. The IgA system may function also to prevent absorption of antigenic material from the gastrointestinal tract. (228) Serums of nearly one-half of patients with IgA deficiency contain precipitating antibodies to milk antigens. (229) A milk allergy is often manifested by persistently loose stools. Apparently, however, not just the colon but the entire gastrointestinal tract is involved in the allergy, as eosinophil counts, the white blood cell that increases in allergies and sensitivities, are found to be higher even in duodenal tissue. (230) It has not yet been demonstrated if feeding dairy milk in early life is the **cause** of the deficiency in antibodies; but it is known that the immune system is injured by too early exposure to animal protein. Milk can permanently injure the gastrointestinal tract, and may be the offending agent in celiac disease, a distressing disease having severe abdominal and general symptoms. Celiac disease is associated with food allergies in about one-third of cases with the injury to the gastrointestinal tract being manifested by atrophic changes in the lining of the small bowel. (231)

When an antigen from an outside source meets an antibody produced by the person, a chemical battle occurs in which the antigen is held in a clinch by the antibody. The clinch is called a complex. Infants given dairy milk have more circulating antigen/antibody complexes than do infants not fed milk. Breast-fed infants have been shown **not to have** circulating antigen/antibody complexes, which are **universal** in dairy formula fed infants! Circulating antigen/antibody complexes are capable of damaging various tissues such as renal tissues, blood vessels and joints, and can interfere with cellular immunity. (232) Such injury may predispose to serious degenerative disease such as arthritis, nephritis, or atherosclerosis later in life. The child with recurrent runny nose and cough will often be relieved entirely of symptoms when milk and its products are eliminated from the diet. (233)

Attempts have been made to modify the manifestations of allergic types of disease in infants by reducing the antigenic exposure during the early months of life. Artificial formula feeding has been incriminated as a possible cause of asthma in infancy. General anesthesia during the first two years of life may predispose to asthma and join with other factors to cause the development of other allergic types of disease. All elective surgery should be avoided during the first two years of life in an effort to lessen the subsequent risk of allergic respiratory disease. (234)

Several cases of occasional bloody urine have been reported to be caused by milk drinking in both adults and children. Bloody urine invariably followed unboiled milk consumption in one child. (235)

A 5-month-old Chinese girl began vomiting blood clots. Her symptoms cleared upon switching her from milk formula to Sobee (a soy preparation), and recurred within 48 hours of a trial feeding with milk. Three such challenges with a test dose of milk were positive, and the symptoms subsided following the discontinuance of milk after each challenge. (236)

FAILURE TO THRIVE, ANEMIA AND RESPIRATORY DISEASE

Six black children were reported to have failure to thrive, anemia, and pulmonary symptoms including wheezing and infiltrates in the lungs by x-ray, enlarged adenoids, and finally right heart failure. They were found to have pulmonary hemosiderosis (deposits of blood pigments in the lungs) because of hyperreactivity to milk. (237)

Three patients with urticaria (hives) were shown to break out with skin lesions if they were fed as little as one-fifth of a teaspoon of milk. (238) For a long time, it has been believed by some investigators that the use of milk formulas is somehow related to crib deaths (or sudden infant death syndrome.) (239)

Connecticut Health Department investigators recently sampled evaporated milks and found that all were contaminated with lead, containing an average of 0.36 ppm. Milk samples from eight women living in the same area had no lead. Hyperactivity in children has been associated with high lead levels in tissue and hair. Hyperactivity is less common in breast-fed infants. Treatment of all cases of hyperactivity in children should begin with removing milk from the diet.

Milk allergy is not confined to childhood or infancy, but is very frequently seen in adults; the commonest type of food allergy in the United States today is milk allergy. In adults we see nasal congestion, hay fever, asthma, middle ear afflictions, croup, headaches, dizziness, seizures, tension, fatigue, constipation, gas, bloating, intestinal noises, diarrhea, abdominal burning and pain, vomiting blood, loss of appetite, colitis, adult bedwetting, blood in the urine, pallor and facial swelling, skin allergies, itching and aching in the musculoskeletal system all associated with milk drinking. The diagnosis of milk allergy can be made at any age, and is often delayed in onset, that is, it does not appear immediately upon drinking the milk or eating food containing dairy products or dairy by-products. It is this particular characteristic of milk allergy that protects it from being suspected when one of the numerous symptoms of milk sensitivity appear in a child. Apart from respiratory tract symptoms, the most frequently seen symptoms and signs of delayed-onset food allergy are probably headache, fatigue, pallor, dark shadows under the eyes, irritability, and stomach ache. (240)

Longstanding painful shoulder has been caused by an allergy to milk and cheese in two patients, twelve years in one and twenty years in the other. Headaches, fuzzy vision, and skin problems were associated symptoms in one of the patients. Cheese was even more capable of producing symptoms than milk. (241) It is quite likely that many obscure symptoms in patients, causing much discomfort and disability, are related to food allergies--milk being the food most suspect as it is responsible for over half of all food sensitivities, all other foods together accounting for only about 40% of sensitivity symptoms.

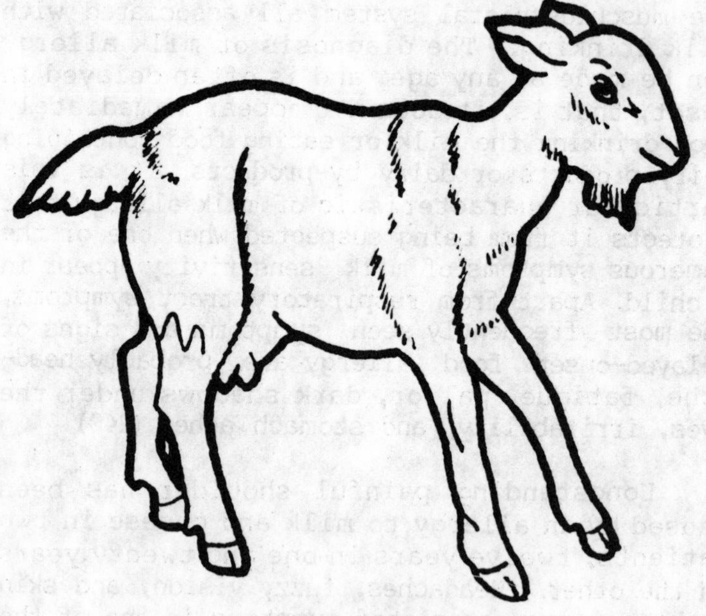

CHAPTER SIXTEEN
Cheese

DECOMPOSITION OF MILK

Cheese is made by coagulating milk, usually with the help of an added coagulant such as rennet; stirring and heating the curd; draining off the whey and collecting or pressing the curd. Then follows a long curing or "ripening" operation, similar to the process of composting leaves, during which the major nutrients undergo a form of decomposition due to the action of bacteria. Factors responsible for nutritional changes in milk used in manufacture of cheese are

1. The method of curd coagulation
2. The extent of whey removed
3. The conditions of the ripening process, such as length, maintenance temperature, types of germs or fungi causing the nutrient decomposition, etc.

After the proteins are coagulated by rennet or lactic acid formed during fermentation by bacteria, the whey is separated. Losses of milk nutrients are greatest in the whey separation stage. One-third of the calcium is lost, 25% of the protein, 75% of riboflavin, 85% of thiamine, 90% of niacin, and about 100% of vitamin C are lost. These losses occur both in hard cheese and in cottage cheese. Cottage and cream cheese contain only 20% of the calcium and phosphorus of the original milk. Any vitamins contributed by the growth of molds is insignificant, since they remain on the surface and are trimmed away.

During the fermentation or curing of cheese, a mixed group of microorganisms grows in the milk curd, affecting the flavor and firmness of the cheese. Protein, fat, and carbohydrate are the major nutrients affected during the curing process. The protein portion of cheese is fermented with the formation of peptides, amines, indoles, skatole, and ammonia. Migraine headaches can be caused by tyramine, one of the amines produced in cheese. Certain of the amines can interact with the nitrites present in the stomach to form nitrosamine, a cancer-producing agent. The fat in cheese is hydrolyzed to irritating fatty acids: butyric, caproic, caprylic, and longer carbon chain fatty acids. Some of the changes that occur in fats and cholesterol upon aging are of a nature as to render them dangerous to health. (242) Three forms of oxidized cholesterol that occur with aging (see page 73) and cause very rapid damage to artery walls may be found in some common foods--lard, ripened cheese, pancake mix, powdered eggs, and custards. One infant formula was shown to contain a type of oxidized cholesterol. One pioneer nutrition writer, Ellen G. White, counselled in 1868, "Cheese should never be introduced into the stomach." (243) Nobody would think of spoiling other foods before eating them; nor does it do anything good for the already questionable wholesomeness of milk to spoil it.

The carbohydrate of milk, mainly lactose, is converted to lactic acid by putrification. Most of the products of fermentation are toxic and irritating, including the esters, the acids, and certain of the amines, such as tyramine and nitrosamine.

RENNET AND RIPENING

The rennet used in the curdling of milk for cheese making is obtained from the whole stomach lining of calves, lambs, kids or pigs. The flesh of the animal's stomach lining is ground, the enzyme contained with the lining being the active portion. Since cottage cheese and cream cheese are not "ripened" it seems reasonable to some that these products can be safely used. They are safe, however, only if free from disease-producing organisms, heavy metals, detergents, antibiotics, cancer viruses, and other undesirable substances found in milk. In this day of expanding diseases in animals, and expanding processes of manufacture and marketing it is highly unlikely that rennet is free from the diseases which can be transmitted from such meat items as steak and pork chops. "Children are allowed to eat flesh meats, spices, butter, cheese, pork, rich pastry, and condiments generally... These things do their work of deranging the stomach, exciting the nerves to unnatural action and enfeebling the intellect." (244)

Cheese washer's disease, a hypersensitivity pneumonia, and "cheese reaction," a characteristic disease of severe hypertension, headache, palpitations, neck pain, and occasional intracranial hemorrhage and heart failure are caused by tyramine and other pressor amines which are natural constituents of ripened cheeses. The disease is much more likely to occur in persons taking an antidepressant. Six patients in which diabetic neuropathy was diagnosed ate cheese and subsequently broke out in severe facial sweating illustrating the influence of the pressor amines on the general body physiology. Chocolate, alcohol, and pickles may also provoke sweating after eating. (245)

POLIO VIRUSES AND CHEDDAR CHEESE

Polio viruses can survive in cheddar cheese throughout the life of the product. Most cheeses are made of unpasteurized milk. Salmonella, Staphylococci, and Brucella organisms can survive long periods in the cheese. A number of outbreaks of disease, as well as food poisoning, have been traced to cheese and milk powder. (246) Enterotoxin A from **Staphylococcus aureus** persisted for over three years in cheddar cheese made with normal or inhibited starter. (247)

In 1947, it was felt that attention should be drawn to lack of control and supervision of the manufacture and sale of cheese. Numerous epidemics in the United States and elsewhere could be traced to it. In the order of incidence, the epidemics were as follows: food poisoning, typhoid, gastroenteritis, diarrhea, and botulism. The situation is not much better today. (248)

CHAPTER SEVENTEEN
Hunger and Appetite as Related to Milk

APPETITE IS CULTIVATED

Hunger and appetite are two entirely different mechanisms of the neurophysiology. The former is a natural instinct, but the latter is an acquired characteristic. Hunger is painful and can be relieved by eating very, very small amounts of food, especially voluminous foods like milk. Appetite is a cultivated characteristic, but its correct development must be accomplished by repeated stimulation from hunger. Occasional hunger is essential to proper development of appetite and its control. Excessive appetite in later childhood or in adulthood can be developed by excessive milk consumption, prolonged hunger, or by early malnutrition. It is our belief that excessive milk drinking in childhood initially depresses the appetite, then encourages a rebound appetite of such large proportions that excessive milk drinking often occurs in these adults, the final outcome being an inordinate craving for milk and milk products.

MILK APPETITE MAY BE AN ALLERGY

The mechanism for the large appetite for milk, according to some of the recently developed theories on food allergies, is that cravings can develop for those things which injure one, and, of course, those foods to which one becomes allergic cause injury to the body. The early feeding of milk is highly likely to be the cause of so much milk sensitivity. Drinking milk in infancy promotes multicell obesity, and may cause the child to have the stage set for his lifelong fight with overweight. To help correct these health and feeding problems, the great curtailment of the use of milk seems a reasonable answer.

APPENDIX A

In the mid-thirties, a virus discovered by Bittner was found in the milk of a cancer-susceptible strain of mice. The tumors could be prevented or greatly reduced in incidence, by taking the offspring of a susceptible strain of mice from the mother immediately after birth and transferring them for nursing to foster mothers of a cancer-resistant strain. The Bittner mouse factor, a heavy particle with "virus-like dimensions" is now recognized to be a cancer virus particle, and the cause of the continuing high incidence of cancer in that strain of mice. It has been shown that males could transmit the virus to virus-free females at mating.

It has long been confirmed that a particular virus causes cancer of the breast in mice. As long ago as 1942 and earlier, investigators have had sufficient evidence to state as follows: "It has been established that an 'influence' contained in the breast milk of mice of high mammary cancer strains is important in determining the development of mammary cancer in these stocks." (109) Since the work in 1942, this 'influence' has been shown to be a virus.

APPENDIX B

Budding "C"-type viral particles have been found in lymphocytes (a type of white blood cell) recovered from the blood of normal and leukemic cattle. Similar viruses have been found in the lymphocytes of dairy milk. Virus-like particles have also been found in milk, in tissue biopsies, and in cell cultures derived from leukemic cows. (113)

APPENDIX C

DOES THE VIRUS CONTROL THE TYPE OF CANCER PRODUCED?

Polyoma virus produces many different types of cancers (salivary gland, breast, kidney, thymus, thyroid, adrenal, and stomach), and affects many different types of laboratory animals (hamster, rat, guinea pig, rabbit, and mouse). The virus can be spread through saliva and body excreta, and is passed vertically through the milk. Laboratory workers who have worked with the virus for long periods show antibodies in their blood. The wart viruses (papilloma) of rabbit, dog, cow, horse, and man are similar in structure, and probably represent an example of one virus infecting different hosts. Human adenovirus has caused adenovirus-type tumors in newborn hamsters, (114) furnishing evidence of the cancer-inducing potential of a human virus. In fact, at least eight of the 31 known human adenoviruses are tumor-inducing in newborn hamsters.

Few researchers doubt any longer that viruses are a primary cause of cancer in man, since transmission of cancer viruses to primates and other mammals have been proven. Virologist Freidrich Deinhardt of St. Luke's Hospital in Chicago said "It would indeed be surprising if the Almighty had made man alone among primates immune to this agent." (169)

BIBLIOGRAPHY

1. The Global Importance of Parasitic Zoonoses. **WHO Chronicle** 34:131-138, 1980

2. Leptospirosis: A Contemporary Zoonosis. **Annals of Internal Medicine** 79:893-894, 1973

3. What Is The Current Status of the Zoonoses? **Journal of Laboratory Medicine** 1:28-33, 1970

4. The Food Vehicle in Virus Transmission. **Health Laboratory Science** 1:51-59, 1964

5. Ibid

6. A Review of Some Animal Diseases Encountered at Meat Inspection. **The Veterinary Record** 87:234-238, 1980

7. Cheese and Its Relation to Disease. **American Journal of Public Health** 37:987-996, 1947

8. Diseases of Children Acquired from Nondomestic Animals. **Current Problems in Pediatrics** 4(10)3-45, August, 1974

9. Frequency of Fish Tumors Found in a Polluted Watershed as Compared to Non-Polluted Canadian Waters. **Cancer Research** 33:189-198, February, 1973

10. GAO: 14% of Meat, Poultry Contains Harmful Residues. **Fort Launderdale News and Sun-Sentinel**, April 22, 1979, p. 4D

11. Drugged Cows: Antibiotics and Feed for Thought. **Time** 114;49, September 10, 1979

12. Immunochemical Resemblance Between Human Leukemia and Hen Egg-White Lysozyme and Their Reduced Carboxymethyl Derivatives. **Journal of Molecular Biology** 61:237-250, October 14, 1971

13. Carcinogenic Activity of the Growth Factor from Egg Yolk and Its Relation to Endogenous Carcinogen. **Neoplasma** (Suppl. 1)98-102, 1960

14. Conjunctival Allergy for Egg Yolks. **Ateno Parmense** 23:1596-1600, 1952

15. Egg White Edema in Rats and Adrenal Activity. **The Journal of Allergy** 24:479-482, 1953

16. Transient Cerebral Ischemia Attacks Related to Egg Consumption. **Postgraduate Medical Journal** 57:642-644, October, 1981

17 Campylobacter Enteritis--Iowa. **Morbidity and Mortality Weekly Reports From the**

Center For Disease Control 28(47)565-566, November 30, 1979

18. One Man's Meat... .**The Sciences** 19:2-3, November, 1979

19. Thermal Resistance of Salmonellae in Egg Yolk Products Containing Sugar or Salt. **Poultry Science** 48:1156-1166, July, 1969

20. Paratyphoid Fever from Frozen Chinese Eggs. **British Medical Journal** 1:1115-1116, May 4, 1963

21. Polychlorinated Biphenyl Exposure--Idaho, Montana. **Morbidity and Mortality Weekly Report From the Center For Disease Control** 28(38)449-450, September 28, 1979

22. Outbreak of Trichinosis--Louisiana. **Morbidity and Mortality Weekly Report from the Center For Disease Control** 28(30)357-358, August 3, 1979

23. Group R Streptococcal Infection Amongst Pig Meat Handlers--A Review. **Public Health** (London) 93:140-142, 1979

24. Hotdogs a Potential Source of Pathogens. **Journal of the American Medical Association** 222(6)633, November 6, 1972

25. Diphyllobothriasis. **American Family Physician** 20(3)127-128, September, 1979

26. Syndrome of Infant Botulism. **Pediatrics**

59:321-322, March, 1977

27. Botulism and Sudden Infant Death Syndrome. **Journal of the American Medical Association** 238:1629, October 10, 1977

28. Some Manifestations of Animal Diseases Transmissible to Man: Pruritis. **Proceedings of the Royal Society of Medicine** 62:1049-1050, October, 1969

29. Food Poisoning and Poisonous Foods. **Emergency Medicine**, October, 1977, p. 195

30. Paratyphoid Fever From Frozen Chinese Eggs. **British Medical Journal** 1:1175-1176, July, 1963

31. Two Outbreaks of Egg-Borne Salmonellosis and Implications for Their Prevention. **Journal of the American Medical Association** 199(6)372-378, February 6, 1967

32. Thermal Resistance of Salmonellae in Egg Yolk Products Containing Sugar or Salt. **Poultry Science** 48:1156-1166, July, 1969

33. Salmonella Gastroenteritis Associated with Milk--Arizona. **Morbidity and Mortality Weekly Report** 28(10)117-120, March 16, 1979

34. Salmonellosis Associated with Consumption of NonFat Powdered Milk--Oregon. **Morbidity and Mortality Weekly Report** 28(11)124-130, March 23, 1979

35. Interstate Outbreak of Salmonella

Newbrunswick Infection Traced to Powdered Milk. **Journal of the American Medical Association** 203(10)838-844, March 4, 1968

36. Salmonella Agona Infection May Be Result of Contact with Riding Horses. **American Journal of Veterinary Research** 40:1301,

37. Diseases from Pets. **The Medical Letter** 15(18)73-75, 1973

38. Salmonellosis in Children from Pet Turtles Certified Salmonella Free. **Clinical Pediatrics** 13(9)719, September, 1974

39. Diseases of Children Acquired from Nondomestic Animals. **Current Problems in Pediatrics** 4(10)3-45, August, 1974

40. Salmonella Carrier May Work as Artificial Inseminator of Turkeys. **Journal of the American Medical Association** 221(10)1172, September 4, 1972

41. Salmonellosis: Report of a Human Case Following Direct Contact with Infected Cattle. **Canadian Medical Association Journal** 96:1163, April 22, 1967

42. Epidemic Yersinia Enterocolitica Infection Due to Contaminated Chocolate Milk. **New England Journal of Medicine** 298(2)76-79, 1978

43. Food Poisoning and Poisonous Foods. **Emergency Medicine**, October, 1977 p. 195-201

44. Milk, Its Relation to Infectious Diseases. **New Orleans Medical and Surgical Journal** 80:11-16, July, 1927

45. Brucellosis in the United States. **Journal of the American Medical Association** 244(20)2318-2322, November 21, 1980

46. Georgia Receives Federal Funds for Brucellosis Eradication. **Farmer's and Consumer's Market Bulletin** 62:1, September 29, 1976

47. Investigacao Da Brucelose Em Bovinos E Em Consumidores Humanos Do Leite. **Rev. Saude Pub. S. Paulo** 11:238-247, 1977

48. Brucellosis in the United States. **Journal of the American Medical Association** 244(20) 2318-2322, November 21, 1980

49. The Role of Milk in the Causation of the Chicago Epidemic of Sore Throat. **Journal of the American Medical Association** 59(19) 1715-1917, November 9, 1912

50. An Epidemic of Sore Throat Due to Milk. **Journal of the American Medical Association** 68(18)1305-1309, May 5, 1917

51. Oski, Frank and J. D. Bell **Don't Drink Your Milk.** Wyden Books, 1977

52. A Strep That Can't Be Trusted. **Emergency Medicine**, May 15, 1979, p. 34-40

53. Pets and Rheumatoid Arthritis. **Arthritis and Rheumatism** 17(3)229, 1974

54. The Primary Cause of Rheumatoid Arthritis Is An Infection--The Infectious Agent Exists in Milk. **Acta Medica Scandinavica** 192:231-239, 1972

55. Oyster Associated Hepatitis. **Journal of the American Medical Association**233:1065, 1975

56. Hepatitis Epidemic Conveyed by Raw Oysters. **Svenska Lakartidningen** 53(16)989, 1956

57. Changing Concepts in the Epidemiology of Viral Hepatitis. **New England Journal of Medicine** 278:1371, June 20, 1968

58. Exotic Newcastle Disease--Why Is the Government Worried About It? **News Feature, United States Department of Agriculture** 2201-2279

59. Investigations on the Variability of Pathogenicity. **Acta Microbiologica Polonica** 14:303-308, 1956

60. Leptospirosis: A Contemporary Zoonosis. **Annals of Internal Medicine** 79:893-894, December, 1973

61. Domestic Pets and Their Relationship to Human Disease. **Royal Society of Health Journal** 87:115-119, March-April, 1967

62. Leptospirosis in Human Pregnancy Followed

by Death of the Fetus. **British Medical Journal** 1:228-229, January 25, 1969

63. Veterinary Workers and Disseminated Sclerosis. **Journal of Neurology, Neurosurgery and Psychiatry** 26:514-515, December, 1963

64. Virus May Cause Dementia of Jakob-Creutzfeldt, Alzheimer's. **Internal Medicine News**, June 15, 1978

65. Fatal Foot-and-Mouth Disease in an Adult Caused by Coxsackievirus A7. **Journal of the American Medical Association** 242(10)1065, September 7, 1979

66. Persistence of Foot-and-Mouth Virus in Butter and Butter Oil. **Journal of Dairy Research** 45:283-285, 1978

67. Current Concepts in Parasitology: Toxocaral Visceral Larva Migrans. **New England Journal of Medicine** 298:436-439, February 23, 1978

68. The Role of House Pets in the Transmission of Diseases of Medical Importance. **Journal of the Phillipine Medical Association** 43:115-121, February, 1967

69. Serologic Diagnosis of Toxocara Canis Infection. **Southern Medical Journal** 73(4) 435-437, April, 1980

70. Listeria Revisited. **American Journal of Diseases of Childhood** 131:391-392, 1977

71. Transmission of Haemorrhagic Disease From Monkeys to Man. **The Lancet** 294:901-902, April 27, 1968

72. Pets, Parasites, and Pediatrics. **Pediatrics** 36(4)521-522, October, 1965

73. Systemic Lupus Erythematosus--A Zoonosis? **Scandanavian Journal of Rheumatology** 8:222-224, 1979

74. Role of Household Animals in Maintenance of Cholera Infection in a Community. **Journal of Infectious Diseases** 130(6)575-579, December, 1974

75. Human Plague--Texas, New Mexico. **Monthly Morbidity and Mortality Report** 30(12):137-138, April 3, 1981

76. Anthrax Infection in Bone Meal From Various Countries of Origin. **Journal of Hygiene** 70:455-457, September, 1972

77. Ambrose, E.J. **The Surface Properties of Mammalian Cells in Culture:** Williams and Wilkins, 1968, p. 23-39

78. Charges on the Cell Membrane. **Science News** 97:312, March 28, 1970

79. Viruses May Repress Contact Inhibition. **Science News** 93:497, May 25, 1968

80 Preliminary Observations on New Lymphoblastic Strains (EB4, EB5) from Burkitt Tumors in a British and Ugandan

Patient. **British Journal of Cancer** 20(3) 475-479, September, 1966

81. Thermal Resistance of Certain Oncogenic Viruses Suspended in Milk and Milk Products. **Applied Microbiology** 22:315-320, September, 1971

82. Virus-Cancer Tie Affirmed by NCI in a Rare Leukemia. **Medical World News,** September 14, 1981, p. 8

83. Viruses and Water Quality. **Journal of the American Medical Association** 219:1628, March 20, 1972

84. Preliminary Observations on New Lymphoblastic Strains (EB4, EB5) from Burkitt Tumors in a British and Ugandan Patient. **British Journal of Cancer** 20(3)475-479, September, 1966

85. Milk-Borne Cancerogenic Virus. **Journal of the American Medical Association** 140(7) 607

86. Cancer of the Breast Linked to Virus in New Evidence. **Medical Tribune,** April 28, 1971, page 1

87. Simian Virus of Breast Cancer Like Others. **Hospital Tribune** 4(9)1, May 4, 1970

88. Titration of the Milk Agent Virus in Milk and Lactating Mammary Gland Cells. **Cancer Research** 10:516-520, August, 1950

89. Viruses and Breast Cancer. **Hospital Practice** 7:72-81, January, 1972

90. Cancer of Breast Linked to Virus in New Evidence. **Medical Tribune** April 28, 1971, page 1

91. More Clout for Human Cancer Viruses. **Science News** 103:121, February 24, 1973

92. Leukemia and Multiple Myeloma in Farmers. **American Journal of Epidemiology** 94:307-310, 1971

93. Virus-Like Particles in Cow's Milk from a Herd with a High Incidence of Lymphosarcoma. **Journal of the National Cancer Institute** 33:2055-1064, 1964

94. Experiments on the Transmission of Bovine Leukosis by Colostrum and Milk. **Bibliotheca Haematologica** 30:146-148, 1968

95. Breast Cancer--Particles in Milk? **CA** 27(1)53, January-February, 1977

96. From Cancerous Cows, Pneumonia. **Medical World News**, May 12, 1972, p. 60

97. Hepatic Tumors in Rats Following the Prolonged Ingestion of Milk and Egg Yolk. **Cancer Research** 14:441-444, July, 1915

98. Leukemia and Multiple Myeloma in Farmers. **American Journal of Epidemiology** 94:307-310, 1971

99. More Clout for Human Cancer Virus. **Science News** 103:121, February 24, 1973

100. Interspecies Transmission of Leukemia Agent Likely. **Antibiotic News,** April 5, 1967, p. 4

101. Beeson, Paul B., M.D. and Walsh McDermott, M.D. **Cecil-Loeb Textbook of Medicine,** 12th Edition, Philadelphia: W. B. Saunders, 1967, p. 1068

102. **Roche Image of Medicine and Research** Spring, 1973

103. Hodgkin's in Ohio: Evidence for Virus? **Science News** 103:85, February 20, 1973

104. Human Leukemia Passed to Animals. **Science News** 91:311, April 1, 1967

105. Oncogenic Transformation of Hamster Cells After Exposure to Herpes Simplex Virus Type 2. **Nature New Biology** 233:48-50, September 8, 1971

106. Interspecies Transmission of Leukemia Agent Likely. **Antibiotic News,** April 5, 1967, p. 4

107. Track of the Cat at Leukemia Scene. **Medical World News,** October 17, 1969, p. 13-14

108. A Household Cluster of Feline Malignant Lymphoma. **Cancer Research** 27:1316-1322, July, 1967

109. Public Health Aspects of Cancer in Pet Dogs and Cats. **American Journal of Public Health** 62:1400-1402, November, 1972

110. Sick Pets and Human Leukemia. **Annals of Internal Medicine,** 78:605, April, 1973

111. Pets and Human Leukemia. **American Journal of Public Health** 62:1520-1531, 1972

112. More Clout for Human Cancer Viruses. **Science News** 103:124, February 24, 1973

113. A Multiple Share of Myeloma. **Medical World News,** May 16, 1969, p. 23

114. What Causes Cancer on the Farm? **Medical World News,** January 14, 1972, p. 39

115. Intestinal Cancer May Be Increased by Meat Ammonia. **Medical Tribune,** September 20, 1972

116. Meat and Fat Consumption and Cancer Mortality. **The Lancet,** 1:946, April 24, 1982

117. A Bowl a Day--Less Stomach CA? **Medical World News,** February 16, 1973, p. 72-73

118. High Birth Weight and Leukemia. **Science News** 100:99, October 9, 1971

119. Alterations in Cell Membrane Linked to All Forms of Cancer. **Medical Tribune,** December 27, 1972

120. Foreign Proteins. **Science News** 89:283, April 23, 1966

121. Ibid

122. Carcinogenic Effect of Hens' Eggs as Part of the Diet in Mice. **Proceedings of the Society for Experimental Biology and Medicine** 102:748-751, 1959

123. Presence of a Carcinogenic Substance in Hens' Eggs. **Proceedings of the Society for Experimental Biology and Medicine** 96:332-335, 1957

124. Cancer: From Fowl to Woman? **Time** 83:79, April 3, 1964

125. **Report of the Regional Poultry Research Laboratory,** E. Lansing, MI. 1949

126. **Life and Health,** October, 1971, p. 34

127. **Report of the Regional Poultry Research Laboratory,** E. Lansing, MI. 1949

128. Diet Helps Children with Acute Leukemia. **Science News** 89:423, May 28, 1966

129. Six of Nine Foods Linked with Bowel Cancer Risks are Meats. **Internal Medicine News,** January 1, 1973

130. Hodgkin's in Ohio: Evidence for Virus? **Science News** 103:85, February 10, 1973

131. Charges on the Cell Membrane. **Science News** 97:312, March 28, 1970

132. Exploring a New Route to Leukemia. **Medical World News,** July 5, 1968, p. 27

133. Dessication of Cells May Trigger Cancer. **Medical World News,** September 10, 1965, p. 49

134. The Effects of Exercise on the Growth of a Mouse Tumor. **Cancer Research** 4:116, February, 1944

135. Mutagens, Carcinogens, and Tumor Promoters in Our Daily Food. **Cancer** 49(10)1970-1984, May 15, 1982

136. Persistence of Health Habits and Their Relationship to Mortality. **Preventive Medicine** 9:469-483, 1980

137. Nutrition Briefs. **Science News** 103:150, March 20, 1973

138. Krause, Marie, M.S., R.D., and Martha Hunscher, B.S., M.Ed., R.D. **Food, Nutrition, and Diet Therapy,** Philadelphia: W. B. Saunders Company, 1972, p. 74

139. The Socio-Cultural Syndrome of Milk. **Journal of Applied Nutrition,** Winter, 1975, p. 6-9

140. Ibid.

141. On the Absence of Cow's Milk from Japan: Its Beneficial Consequences. **Journal of the American Medical Association** 20(4):83, January 28, 1893

142. Nutrition and Vegetarianism. **Dairy Council Digest** 50(1), January-February, 1979

143. The Nutritional Adequacy of a Vegetable Substitute for Milk. **British Journal of Nutrition** 5:269-274, 1951

144. Ibid

145. The Role of Dairy Foods in Diet. **Dairy Council Digest** 48(3)14, May-June, 1977

146. Dietary Factors in Dental Decay. **Nutrition and the M.D.** 2(12)1, May, 1979

147. Calcium to Phosphorus Ratios. **Contemporary Nutrition** 4(5)1, May, 1979

148. Altschule, Mark D. **Nutritional Factors in General Medicine.** Springfield: C. C. Thomas, 1978, p. 163

149. White, Ellen G. **The Ministry of Healing** Mountain View, CA: Pacific Press Publishing Company, 1942, p. 321

150. Overuse of Milk in the Diets of Infants and Children. **Journal of the American Medical Association** 172(6)567-569, February 6, 1960

151. Hyperreactivity to Cow's Milk in Young

Children with Pulmonary Hemosiderosis and Cor Pulmonale Secondary to Nasopharyngeal Obstruction. **The Journal of Pediatrics** 87(1)23-29, July, 1975

152. You Can Add Cow's Milk to Hazardous Food List, Doctor Says. **Sun-Sentinel,** January 18, 1979

153. Filled Milks, Imitation Milks, and Coffee Whiteners. **Pediatrics** 49:770-775, May, 1972

154. White, Ellen G. **Counsels on Diet and Foods** Takoma Park, Washington D. C.: Review and Herald Publishing Association, 1946, p. 411

155. Ibid. p. 414

156. Ibid. p. 359

157. The Role of the Combination of Sucrose and Milk Products in Diabetes Mellitus and Ischemic Heart Disease. **Medical Hypothesis** 1:191, September-October, 1975

158. Role of the Combination of Sucrose and Milk in Diabetes Mellitus. **American Journal of Clinical Nutrition** 31(4)559-560, April, 1978

159. Dietary Carbohydrate and Serum Cholesterol Levels in Man. **American Journal of Clinical Nutrition** 18:237, 1966

160. Role of the Combination of Sucrose and Milk in Diabetes Mellitus. **American Journal of**

Clinical Nutrition 31(4)559-560, April, 1978

161. Milk Has Something For Everybody? **Journal of the American Medical Association** 232(5) 539, May 5, 1975

162. Some Diseases of Cattle Transmitted to Man Through Milk. **Journal of the American Veterinary Medical Association** 78:500-505, 1931

163. Mills, Lewis Craig, M.D. and John H. Moyer, M.D. **Shock and Hypotension,** New York: Grune and Stratton Publishers, 1965

164. Infants--Even Fetuses--Show Pre-atherosclerotic Lesions. **Medical Tribune,** October 5, 1977, p. 2

165. Milk Has Lowering Effect on Blood Serum Cholesterol. **Nutrition Notes 77,** Fall, 1978, p. 8

166. Serum Cholesterol Levels of Mexican and Wisconsin School Children. **American Journal of Epidemiology** 96:36-39, July, 1972

167. Spontaneously Occurring Angiotoxic Derivatives of Cholesterol. **American Journal of Clinical Nutrition,** 32:40-47, 1979

168. Ibid

169. Track of the Cat At Leukemia Scene **Medical World News** October 17, 1969, p. 13, 14

170. Food Allergy Is Seen As Producing Pulmonary Disease. **Internal Medicine News,** January 15, 1977

171. Milk Protein and Other Food Antigens in Atheroma and Coronary Heart Disease. **American Heart Journal** 81:289, February, 1971

172. Further Evidence in the Case Against Heated Milk Protein. **Atherosclerosis** 15:129, January-February, 1972

173. Dangers of a High Protein Diet. **Science News** 103:271, April 18, 1971

174. The Case Against Heated Milk Protein. **Atherosclerosis** 13:137-139, January-February, 1971

175. Postprandial Drowsiness. **Journal of the American Medical Association** 220:1135, May 22, 1972

176. Leucine Sensitive Hypoglycemia. **Jewish Hospital Bulletin,** March, 1969, p. 63-69

177. Briggs,George M., Ph.D., and Doris H. Calloway, Ph.D. **Bogert's Nutrition and Physical Fitness** 10th Edition, 1979, p. 294

178. Current Concepts in Infant Nutrition. **Dairy Council Digest** 37(2)10, March-April, 1976

179. Krause, Marie. **Food, Nutrition, and Diet**

Therapy, Philadelphia: W. B. Saunders, 1972, p. 127

180. Acrodermatitis Enteropathica, Zinc and Human Milk. **Nutrition Reviews** 36(8)241, 1978

181. Zinc Content of Selected Foods. **Journal of the American Dietetic Association** 66(4):345-355, April, 1975

182. Wohl, Michael, M.D. and Robert S. Goodhart, M.D., **Modern Nutrition in Health and Disease** Philadelphia: Lea and Febieger, 1968, p. 387

183. Zinc, A Lifesaver for AE Babies. **Medical World News**, October 25, 1974, p. 39

184. CAD Rate Low Where Milk is Ultrapasteurized or Boiled. **Medical Tribune** August 23, 1978

185. Ibid.

186. Correlation of Dairy Food Intake With Human Antibody to Bovine Milk Xanthine. **Proceedings of the Society for Experimental Biology and Medicine,** 160(4)477-482, April, 1979

187. Is Milk A Menace? **Herald of Health,** November 1977, p. 3

188. Milk Protein and Other Food Antigens in Atheroma and Coronary Heart Disease. **American Heart Journal** 81:189, February, 1971

189. Antibiotics in Animal Feeds: Threat to Human Health? **Science News** 101:348-349, May 27, 1972

190. Milk Ups Lead Absorption. **Science News** 119:5, January 3, 1981

191. Cardiovascular Disease Death is Tied to Intake of Cadmium. **Medical Tribune** June, 1972, p. 22

192. Zirconium 95 in Utah Vegetation Produced During the 1966 Growing Season. **Radiological Health Data and Reports,** June, 1970, p. 280

193. The Strontium Spector Again. **Hospital Practice,** 13:144-146, January, 1978

194. Chemical Toxins in Mother's Milk. **Science News** 110:151, September 4, 1976

195. PCBs in Cow's Milk. **Science News** 101:345, May 27, 1972

196. PBBs: More Effects and More Exposure. Science News 112:100-101, August 13, 1977

197. Carcinogenic and Mutagenic Activities of Milk From Cows Fed Bracken Fern. **Cancer Research** 38:1556-1560, June, 1978

198. Excretion of Aflatoxin in a Lactating Cow. **Food and Cosmetic Toxicology** 6:619-625, 1968

199. A Goitrogenic Factor in Milk. **Medical Journal of Australia** 2:645-646, November 2, 1957

200. Calcium as a Goitrogen. **Journal of Clinical Endocrinology** 14:1412-1422, November, 1954

201. A Thyroid-Blocking Agent in the Etiology of Endemic Goiter. **Metabolism** 5:623, 1956

202. Man-Made Maladies and Medicine. **California Medicine** 113:48-53, November, 1970

203. Chronic Rectal Bleeding Due to Milk. **British Medical Journal** 1:1416, 1955

204. Treating the Patient Who Has Chronic Ulcerative Colitis. **Modern Medicine** 44(3) 66-71, February 1, 1975

205. Tidbits and Morsels. **Nutrition and the M.D.** 2(12)4, October, 1976

206. Hypercalcemia and Renal Impairment Following Milk and Alkali Therapy for Peptic Ulcer. **Southern Medical Journal** 48:126-129, February, 1955

207. Unrecognized Disorders Frequently Occurring Among Infants and Children From The Ill Effects of Milk. **Southern Medical Journal** 31:1016, September, 1938

208. Absence of Milk Antibodies in Milk Intolerance in Adults. **Journal of the American Medical Association** 201(2)50,

July 3, 1967

209. Enuresis Treated with A Milk-Free Diet. **Clinical Trends in Family Practice** September-October, 1978, p. 6

210. Diet and the Geographical Distribution of Multiple Sclerosis. **The Lancet** 2:1061 November 2, 1974

211. Cow's Milk As A Cause of Infantile Colic in Breast-Fed Infants. **The Lancet** 2:437-439, August 26, 1978

212. When a Child Has Repeated Colds Think of Milk Allergy. **Consultant**, January, 1968, p. 41

213. Food Allergy: The 10 Common Offenders. **American Family Physician** 13(2)106-112, February, 1976

214. Food Allergy is Seen as Producing Pulmonary Disease. **Internal Medicine News**, January 15, 1977, p. 26

215. Hypertension, Salt Intake, and the Infant. **Postgraduate Medicine** 45:229-230, 1969

216. Cow's Milk Intolerance and Melena. **European Journal of Pediatrics** 132:213-214, 1979

217. **Practical Gastroenterology** 4(7)16, July-August, 1980

218. Colitis, Persistent Diarrhea and Soy

Protein Intolerance. **Journal of Pediatrics** 91:404-407, September, 1977

219. Cow's Milk Protein Sensitive Enteropathy. **Archives of Disease in Childhood** 54:39-43, 1979

220. Psychologic Factors in Milk Anemia. **American Family Physician** 7:80-86, January, 1973

221. Milk as Obstipant. **Journal of the American Medical Association** 230(4)538-539, October 28, 1974

222. Add Milk to Your GI Suspect List. **Patient Care** February 15, 1976, p. 116-126

223. Recurrent Abdominal Pain in Children: Lactose and Sucrose Intolerance, A Prospective Study. **Pediatrics** 64:43-45, July, 1979

224. The Socio-Cultural Syndrome of Milk. **Journal of Applied Nutrition** Winter, 1975, p. 6-9

225. Recognition of Lactose Intolerance. **Hospital Practice** 11:97, October, 1976

226. School Milk Programs Called of Doubtful Value to Blacks. **Medical Tribune,** November 17, 1971, p. 10

227. Cow's Milk-Sensitive Enteropathy. **Archives of Disease in Childhood** 53:375-380, 1978

228. IgA Deficiency and Milk Precipitins. **The Lancet** 1:278, February 6, 1971

229. Antibody to Bovine Milk Common in IgA Deficiency. **Family Practice News** 9(12)59, June 15, 1979

230. Eosinophil Counts In Duodenal Tissue in Cow's Milk Allergy. **The Lancet** 2:361, August 18, 1979

231. Gastrointestinal Allergy and the Celiac Syndrome With Particular Reference to Allergy to Cow's Milk. **Annals of Allergy** 11:426-434, 1953

232. Circulating Immune Complexes in Infants Fed on Cow's Milk. **Nature** 272:632, April 13, 1978

233. Familial Recurrent Rhinorrhea and Bronchitis Due to Cow's Milk. **Journal of the American Medical Association** 198(6)137, November 7, 1966

234. Management of Infantile Asthma. **Southern Medical Journal** 70(9)1055-1058, September, 1977

235. Allergic Hematuria Due to Milk. **New Orleans Medical and Scientific Journal** 101:419-421, March, 1949

236. Milk Allergy and Haemetemesis. **Singapore Medical Journal** 11(2)80-85, June, 1970

237. Hyperreactivity to Cow's Milk in Young

Children with Pulmonary Hemosiderosis and Cor Pulmonale Secondary to Nasopharyngeal Obstruction. **Journal of Pediatrics** 87(1)23-29, July, 1975

238. Complement Activation After Milk Feeding in Children with Cow's Milk Allergy. **The Lancet** 2:893, October 31, 1970

239. Sensibilization of Guinea Pigs With Cow's Milk as a Model of Sudden Death in Infants and Children. **Acta Universitatis Cabolinae Medica** 13(3)207-213, 1967

240. Cow's Milk Allergy: A Critical Review. **Journal of Family Practice** 9(2)223-232, 1979

241. Polymorphic Allergy from Sensitization to Milk and Cheese. **Prensa Medical Argentina** 37:1359, June 23, 1950

242. Spontaneously Occuring Angiotoxic Derivatives of Cholesterol. **American Journal of Clinical Nutrition** 32:40-47, 1979

243. White, Ellen G. **Counsels on Diet and Foods** Takoma Park: Washington D.C.: Review and Herald Publishing Association, 1946, p. 386

244. Ibid. P. 350

245. By the Sweat of Thy Brow. **Journal of the American Medical Association** 232(13)1360, June 30, 1975

246. Cheddar Cheese as a Vehicle for Viruses. **Journal of Dairy Science** 56(10)1329-1331

247. Production of Staphylococcal Enterotoxin A in Cheddar and Colby Cheeses. **Journal of Dairy Science** 54(6)815-825

248. Careful With the Goat's Milk. **Science News** 120:392, December 19 and 26, 1981

INDEX

OTHER BOOKS OF INTEREST

HOME REMEDIES: HYDROTHERAPY, MASSAGE, CHARCOAL, AND OTHER SIMPLE TREATMENTS by Agatha M. Thrash, M.D. and Calvin L. Thrash, Jr. M.D.

An encyclopedia of home remedies ranging from the use of water to treat illness to massage. Clear, easy-to-follow directions guide in treating specific diseases. Emphasis is on common ailments, and arrangement by illness is convenient. The easy-to-read style, simple, non-technical explanations will be appreciated by any reader. $8.95

NUTRITION FOR VEGETARIANS by Agatha M. Thrash, M.D. and Calvin L. Thrash, Jr. M.D.

Nutrition for Vegetarians is a common-sense guide to nutrition for good health. It contains hundreds of up-to-date facts on every phase of nutrition. $8.95

EAT FOR STRENGTH (Regular or Oil-Free Edition)

Over 200 pages packed with a large selection of salads, entrees, dairy product substitutes, desserts and much more. **Eat For Strength** shows that it is possible to eat both wisely and well, and to enjoy the process! $5.95

NATURAL REMEDIES: A MANUAL

A guide to treating over 50 diseases using natural methods.